Endorsements for
You're Not Too Old,
and It's Not Too

"Wonderfully written, You're Not Too Old, and It's Not Too Late offers sage advice and practical exercises to enhance awareness, increase appreciation, bolster resiliency, and boost vitality as we navigate personal challenges and life experiences. Readers of all ages will undoubtedly find something useful in this collection of inspirational stories and research-informed findings."

-Joseph P. Green, Ph.D., Professor of Psychology and Clinical Psychologist, Co-Author of Cognitive-behavioral Therapy, Mindfulness, and Hypnosis for Smoking Cessation: A Scientifically Informed Intervention

"I have found that, as we get older, the challenges of personally navigating the maze of life can be enhanced with these weekly tips from the empathetic and savvy Ilene Berns-Zare."

-Raymond Benson, author of James Bond: the Raymond Benson Years

"This is a delightful book to dip in and out of at leisure. Dr Ilene Berns-Zare has provided an abundance of evidence-informed practices to help manage stress, increase resilience, and cultivate wellbeing in mid-life."

-Claire Higgins, Chief Operating Officer, Positive Psychology Guild

"You're Not Too Old" is a warm and loving invitation to join the author in her daily immersion in and enjoyment of living. Readers will quickly realize that the book title belies an approach to self-care and development that is applicable to ALL stages of adulthood and that charting a path through life can be easier with the right companion. "You're Not Too Old" can be that companion.

-Stephen A. Lisman, Ph.D., SUNY Distinguished Teaching Professor Emeritus (Psychology), Fellow of the Center for Learning and Teaching

"Aging gracefully requires facing many challenges. Fortunately, we do not have to face them alone. In this gem of a book Ilene Berns-Zare combines practical wisdom with insights from positive psychology to create weekly reflections and mindfulness exercises written in a succinct, accessible form. You're Not Too Old is a welcome companion on the journey through midlife and the golden years."

-Thomas R. Mockaitis, Ph.D., Professor of History, DePaul University

"Midlife through older adulthood presents each person with critical opportunities to invigorate their lives, seeking meaning and transformative change. Those choosing a path of more joy, resilience, and fulfillment will find a valuable companion in Dr. Berns-Zare's deft integration of wisdom and science. I love the idea of 52 weeks. It makes the invitation to empower oneself feel so doable."

- Gayle Scroggs, Ph.D., PCC, Women's Paths to Happiness

You're Not Too Old, and It's Not Too Late

Weekly Practices for Meaning, Mindfulness
& New Possibilities at Midlife and Beyond

Ilene Berns-Zare, PsyD

For information, contact
MSI Press
1760-F Airline Highway, #203
Hollister, CA 95023

Copyediting: Betty Lou Leaver
Book layout and cover design: Opeyemi Ikborije

ISBN: 978-1-957354-95-8
LCCN: 2026902261

Some materials reproduced with permission from publications of the author in *Psychology Today*.

Disclaimer: This publication is for informational purposes only. No content is a substitute for consulting with a qualified mental health or healthcare professional. Although the publication is designed to provide accurate information regarding the content, the publisher and the author assume no responsibility for errors, inaccuracies, omissions, or any other inconsistencies herein.

Dedication

This book is dedicated to my husband, Ed Zare, for his ongoing loving support, and to all of you who are and will be seeking greater meaning, resilience, and flourishing in the second half of life.

May love light the way!

CONTENTS

Acknowledgements
with Gratitude

Most everything about this book emerged from a wellspring of experiences, energies, and connections with others. I want to express my heartfelt and expansive gratitude to all who have accompanied me on this meandering, meaningful journey, including all my "teachers" past and present. You have come in many ways—family, friends, family of friends, coaches, mentors, students, and communities.

Ed Zare, you walked me home on a sunny, fall day a long time ago and continue to accompany me, supporting whatever I do, honoring my possibilities, and providing your love so that I can continue to work, play, and grow. You have my deep gratitude for your ongoing presence, trustworthiness, and support. I love you.

Lisa, Julie, Kyle, Sam, Connor, Caylee, Matilda, and Asa—my beloveds. You inspire me not only to stay in shape (parenting and grandparenting flourish with lots of energy) but also to love greatly. Your presence in my world invigorates me to make meaningful, positive contributions that I hope might somehow offer inspiration as you live your own precious lives. May each of you be blessed in all ways, always.

My mom and dad, Muriel Morgan Berns and Frank Berns, both of blessed memories, passed on before this book was published. You carried me before and after I emerged into the world and inspired a push and pull in my life that has motivated me to love, learn, understand, and discover my place in this world. Writing this book in the later chapters of your lives has brought nuanced light and shadow to this journey.

Gail Haller, over these many years you have consistently believed in me and that matters so much. I'll always remember when we used to read my poems, and you truly listened. My heart speaks to your heart.

Bernadette Goheen Kohn, you have inspired my wellspring and whispered to my soul. Ideas for this book may not have emerged without our spiritual sisterhood, which has awakened me to further explore nature's interconnectedness and the nuances of life's energies and melodies.

I am enormously grateful to many people. Steven Jay Lynn, of blessed memory, and Fern Pritikin Lynn offered encouragement, guidance, and support from the beginning and throughout the project. Thank you to Martha Ross-Mockaitis, Tom Mockaitis, Diane Dreher, Toby Lou Hayman, Barbara Stefani, Robert Kohn, Tova Kohn, Lisa Bellows, Nina Mizrahi, Ilana Axel, Ben Dean, Gayle Scroggs, Irene Nizzero, Anne Burman, Nate Ruben, Hannah Ruben, and Roberta (Mickey) Capsuto, of blessed memory, for sharing your support in many different and meaningful ways along this journey.

Thank you to the Wednesday morning class I facilitate each month. I appreciate each of you. To my teachers, colleagues, clients, and friends, I continue to learn, grow, and gain insight from all you share with me. And to all of you who read my articles and who have participated in seminars, webinars, and classes I have offered, I thank you.

I am grateful to Rainer Maria Rilke, who over a century ago reminded us in *Letters to a Young Poet* that "You are not too old, and it is not too late to dive into your increasing depths where life calmly gives out its own secret."

Some material in this book was previously published at *Psychology Today* in my blog: *Flourish and Thrive: Navigating Transitions with Mindfulness and Resilience*. I want to sincerely thank *Psychology Today* Executive Editor, Lybi Ma, who accepted me as blogger in 2018 and Abigail Fagan, my editor, along with the *Psychology Today* editorial team.

Finally, this book would not have been published without the affirmation, support, and editorial guidance of Betty Lou Leaver, managing editor of MSI Press. I am deeply grateful to her for this opportunity. Thank you also to Opeyemi Ikborije for book layout and cover design and to the MSI Press support staff!

To the infinite source that connects us all, may love light the way.

Introduction

Welcome to this journey toward flourishing and resilience at midlife and beyond!

You might think this book is for someone else, someone getting older. And then you realize that someone is *you*. Here, in the 21st century you are not alone. There is unprecedented interest in figuring out how to live well in the middle and later seasons of our lives. We might assume we'll grow wiser by simply adding years. Yet, as most of us meander through young adulthood, middle age, and older adulthood, that's not quite the way it happens.

From ground-breaking discoveries in recent decades, you can learn new practices to help you make the most of your life in each decade. While there's no magic formula, here's an empowering secret: resilience, vitality, and transformative possibilities are nourished with inspiration, information, effort, and resources. You'll learn more about these resources in this book.

As we navigate each stage of our lives, while we have little control over most events outside of ourselves, we *do* have choices about where we direct our attention and the attitudes we bring to our experiences. Our choices can diminish the flow of our resilience and wellbeing or can invigorate mind, body, and spirit.

From young adulthood, through midlife, and into today, I have found companionship by reading inspirational books. My daily readings open windows to other ways to be in the world. Sometimes, studying just a few sentences touches my heart, mind, and spirit in ways that help me shift toward contemplation, new understandings, and actions. These inspirational books often awaken me to moments of mindfulness, wholeness, and new possibilities.

Admittedly, I've not always found life an easy road. If you had asked me 20 years ago whether I would be writing a book about flourishing and resilience, I probably would have shaken my head and laughed. Awakening each morning on the resilient side of the bed is sometimes a challenge. It can take me an hour or more to shift from the shadows of morning light to a more comfortable level of productivity, positivity, and action for the rest of the day. An inspirational book at my side often stirs my motivation to move forward.

During my early adulthood, I questioned the common belief that seeking happiness is one of life's most significant goals. For me, aiming toward a life well-lived had long been about seeking fulfillment, what Viktor Frankl (1985) termed "the search for meaning. In my own experience, engaging in what felt most meaningful brought me the greatest happiness. This seemed to contrast with the understandings of others. I recall telling friends that what was meaningful made me happy and seeing their puzzled reactions. Their responses seemed to say "just go have fun."

In my personal search for meaning, I went on to earn advanced academic degrees, worked in business, education, and wellness, and engaged in personal spiritual and mindfulness practices. Then positive psychology came charging full speed into my life. I studied the work of researchers, including Martin Seligman, Carol Dweck, Ryan Niemiec, and Barbara Fredrickson, noting their findings on happiness, meaningfulness, and well-being. Then, I participated in a professional coach training program (MentorCoach, LLC). Building on these foundations, I began to discern how meaning, wellbeing, and happiness could fit together.

Ideas from my own experience, along with understandings drawn from research on positive psychology and resilience began to converge on many levels. I expanded my understandings about how relationships, positive emotions, meaning, mindfulness, and character strengths can improve the quality of our lives, helping individuals, organizations, and communities flourish.

I've also learned that growing older and aging well are quite different than they used to be. Average life expectancy in developing countries has increased significantly. More than at any previous time in history, we have greater opportunities to shape our own individual aging process—our thoughts, choices, behaviors, and possibilities. We can acknowledge the challenges we encounter at various stages of life while also embracing opportunities for renewing our resilience, reinventing ourselves, and waking up to a more positive narrative about our own lives and possibilities.

How do *you* see the seasons of your life? The paths from young adulthood to midlife to older adulthood are infused with unique blendings of wholeness and vulnerability, clarity and confusion, resilience and resignation, meaning and meaninglessness, light and darkness. Each of us has gifts to share. Life's circumstances offer a myriad of opportunities for nurturing our integral well-being and being intentional about how we relate to the world. Twenty-first century research on adult development invites us to revise how we view adulthood, the questions we ask and respond to, and our own stories as we navigate midlife and the process of growing older.

I hope this book offers you an empowering companion—a reinvigorated, research-informed approach to help you re-map the changing seasons of your adult life. As you move through this volume, you will find many practices that can help you explore and invigorate your well-being, resilience, and happiness.

As you read, I invite you to consider your own perspectives, to re-examine your assumptions about the process of growing older. Consider shedding some of the negative viewpoints that you may be carrying and trying on some new ideas. As you face all that your life serves up, the gifts and the challenges, you can strengthen your capacity for greater joy, meaning, and well-being in your day-to-day existence.

I look forward to sharing this transformational journey with you.

Ilene Berns-Zare

How to Get the
Most from This Book

You're Not Too Old and It's Not Too Late is an invitation to reimagine possibilities for the second half of life in a way that feels right for *you*. Whether you feel you know yourself well or not, these concepts and practices can empower you to transform your ideas about growing older.

The book can be a 52-week companion on your own personal journey. As you read, I hope you will discover vibrant pathways toward personal discovery, adventure, greater freedom, and renewal. Each chapter invites you to awaken to new possibilities for more vibrantly, wholeheartedly, and resiliently navigating the process of growing older, to grow more fully toward becoming your best self in this season of your life.

There are many ways to enjoy this book. Although you can read it cover to cover, a more reflective journey may bring you greater benefits. I recommend that you read a chapter each week, reflecting on the ideas and new insights as you go about your days. Taking it at a comfortable pace, reading and thinking about one chapter at a time may enable the concepts and inspirational nuggets to simmer with your unique personal insights and experiences.

As you begin each week, read a chapter and consider how its content resonates for you. Notice what ideas and strategies catch your interest. Which do you want to experiment with further? Which do you want to incorporate into your life? The choices are up to you.

Some people may prefer to read the book cover to cover first and then choose chapters to delve into more deeply, according to their interests.

Others might enjoy opening the book to a random page and just reading there. Or you may want to choose one chapter that "feels right" to explore.

Consider setting aside time each day to read and reflect on the ideas and inspirations you find. Morning or evening works well for many people. The conclusion of each chapter offers closing inspirations to consider, "*This week I will...*," inviting you to think about ways to apply what you've read about. You might ask yourself: What inspires me? What do I want to reflect on further? How might I experiment with this idea? What's my next right step? When will I do it? What might be changing for me from this practice?

You might choose to record your reflections in a journal, notebook, on your electronic device, or talking into a speech text program. You don't need to write a lot. Even if you write for two minutes, and you're thinking about it, it matters (Pennebaker, 2016). Writing, even very briefly, can help you become more engaged with the content of the book and your own experiences.

One way to get more from this book and take your journey farther is to form a discussion group with a friend or a group of peers. Many people enjoy sharing their reading, thoughts, and experiences with others. One idea is to create a book group or flourishing circle, a discussion group of friends or acquaintances, perhaps meeting weekly or bi-weekly, in-person or virtually, to discuss a chapter, and share the thoughts, questions, and ideas that you're learning and reflecting on. There's something wonderful about sharing your journey with others.

I believe that it's up to us to do the work—it doesn't just happen—as we journey toward flourishing in the second half of life. I hope this book will be a welcome companion, offering meaningful and inspirational ideas, skills, and practices for resilience and flourishing in this season of life.

Come with me now as we begin the journey. May inspiration, wellbeing, and new possibilities light your way!

CHAPTER 1

Welcome to the Journey:
Reimagining Midlife and Beyond

The ideas for this book began to emerge when I was facilitating seminars with adults at midlife and beyond. And okay, I was beginning to kick and scream myself as I thought about how I would do this thing called getting older. Truth be told, as I gazed ahead, what I'd observed happening to *other* people began to feel more real to *me* as I noticed my life had advanced a decade into my 50's, and then suddenly, inexplicably into my 60's.

You're Not Too Old and It's Not Too Late is about engaging the changing seasons of our lives through a kinder, more positive, more courageous lens. Living with this kind of resilience is not a once-and-done choice but a process of realizations, understandings, and choices.

Re-envisioning how we engage with the process of getting older may seem like we need to be superheroes. I don't think this is the case. We can fill our life toolboxes with strategies that can help us steady and strengthen ourselves as we grow older, including daily practices that inspire and empower us.

Many of us are interested in gaining fuller understandings about how to live the best lives we can at any stage—learning strategies to thrive in the face of our vulnerabilities and whatever life throws at us. In my seminars and workshops, I notice people's eyes lighting up as I share information about the importance of finding meaning in our lives, the benefits of relationships, and the advantages of a growth mindset, mindfulness, and engaging our strengths. Sure, we will encounter obstacles as life unfolds and our bodies age, but we have choices about how to respond. We can ask ourselves: "What inspires me? "What can I learn from researchers and experts?" "What strategies can help me live with greater inspiration, courage, and flourishing?"

Navigating midlife and beyond in the 21st century is *not* the same story it was for our parents. New understandings and changes in the ways people live are inviting us to reimagine our ideas about getting older, literally transforming the stories of our lives, moment by moment, as we travel from young adulthood to elderhood.

A growing body of research illustrates that many adults today are healthier and living longer than in the past (Arnett et al., 2020; Institute for Health Metrics and Evaluation, 2024). Adult life transitions occur later in the lifecycle than for previous generations, such as shifting from adolescence to the launch of early adulthood, entering into stable work, joining committed relationships, and becoming parents.

It is not simply that people are living longer. The quality of life in developed countries has changed. Declines as individuals age are not as inevitable as once thought (Diehl et al., 2020). It's becoming clearer that our choices and behaviors can positively impact our future as we grow into elderhood. According to researchers, although genetics is a factor, its influence is often overestimated. We now know that behaviors and changes in behaviors can affect cognitive, physical, and psychological factors that impact our health and well-being (Diehl et al., 2020; Tucker-Drob & Briley, 2014). For example, eating a healthy diet, performing regular physical activity, sharing positive relationships, being open to new ideas, and engaging in activities that use our brains in new and active ways can improve our chances for greater flourishing in the second half of life.

Evidence also indicates that many age-related losses can be delayed, minimized, or even reversed (Diehl et al., 2020; Gill et al., 2009). Looking at growing older through this lens offers a liberating new perspective to redefine the challenges that confront us. This opens opportunities for a greater sense of *agency*, understanding that our actions can make a difference.

This journey may require us to let go of some ways we think about our travels through life. The ideas shared in this book are not intended to ignore the challenges of getting older. Rather, they invite you to reimagine and rewire your understandings and actions, expanding your personal narrative to embrace broader opportunities and possibilities as you travel the winding pathways from young adulthood to elderhood. It is an honor to walk this journey at your side.

Inspirations

As you begin reimagining your journey this week, consider the stories you've been telling yourself about getting older.

To expose your thoughts to the light of day, you might write or draw them in a journal or on a document in your electronic device. Pay attention to the feelings, sensations, and ideas that arise. What are you noticing? Which thoughts and feelings do you want to hold on to? Which aspects of the stories might you want to challenge in the light of new information and a more positive view of midlife and beyond? Perhaps you might consider that the gifts and challenges of your evolving adulthood also expand the fullness of opportunities, grace, and possibilities.

Are you really too old? Is it really too late to shift in some way toward what really matters to you? What current understandings about your emerging story would you like to re-balance or change? What would you like to loosen your ties with or release?

This week I will notice the stories I tell myself about getting older and begin redefining my second half of life.

CHAPTER 2

Rewiring and Re-envisioning
What's Next

I am writing this chapter on Mother's Day during the COVID-19 pandemic while my husband contemplates the process of retiring. In these uncertain times, I feel quite unsettled. Transitions, changes, and losses are filled with significance as I inhabit my personal micro-universe along with a poignant awareness of the ongoing, multi-faceted challenges in our world. I'm concerned about losses of freedoms I once took for granted, and the loss of life so many are dealing with. I am fortunate so far. My loved ones are healthy and well, but I surely miss them—my beloved circle of family and friends.

A huge question hangs in the air. A question I'm trying very hard *not* to notice. Yet, it looms large like a big black bear foraging in the backyard of my midwestern home. What actually stands between what is commonly termed "retirement" and my next chapter in this lifetime? And how can this process and other life transitions be viewed in more expansive ways that affirm what is meaningful in life?

It feels as if I'm standing before a chain link fence, a barrier between "here" and what I've imagined adulthood and elderhood to be. What do I actually know about growing older? What are the truths amid all the stereotypes? Can our vision about growing older be reimagined to take a road less traveled? How strong and resilient is the fence as midlife marches toward older adulthood and beyond?

In the light of day, letting myself notice and turn *toward* rather than away from these uncomfortable questions feels comforting in some way. As I ponder life from this vantage point, I recall that labeling our feelings and thoughts, even the difficult ones, can help us cope more effectively with life's challenges. This pause adds an element of mindful noticing with a kinder lens as I peek hesitantly through the fence. What *could* successful aging look like through a wider, more meaningful lens? Perhaps the more powerfully inspiring question is not "Who am I" and "What will I be transitioning or retiring from", but rather "Who am I becoming?" and "What will I be transitioning toward?"

Holding negative labels and images about older adulthood can reduce our openness to new experiences (Levy, 2009). It is important to be aware of our preconceived ideas about the changing seasons of our lives. With knowledge comes power, as we recognize the assumptions we have been carrying. We can choose to modify unhelpful thoughts and let them go as we reimagine and rewire possibilities for what's next.

Recent findings indicate that we have greater influence to shape our lives as we get older than we once thought (Diehl et al., 2020; Staudinger, 2020). This new research takes into account individual differences, resources, environments, and other circumstances. It opens possibilities to expand and shift self-imposed and societally imposed limitations as we reimagine what's next. Perhaps the cliff is not what I think it is, and perhaps beyond the fence there are other paths to explore for meaning, hope, and calls to action.

My thoughts go to my hero, Dr. Viktor Frankl, renowned psychiatrist and Holocaust survivor, who explained that we have the freedom to choose our attitude between what happens and how we respond (Frankl, 1959). Frankl's life trajectory taught him that with choices come possibilities to search for meaning.

Where and how can we find meaning in the second half of life? One way is to be open to new experiences (Staudinger, 2020). This may involve flexibility and motivation to engage in new and varied activities, such as adventures in learning, personal development, relationships, physical exercise, and new work tasks. Making these kinds of choices can enhance resilience and our capacities to grow in positive ways (Luchetti et al., 2016; Staudinger, 2020)

Creativity in this season of our lives is another piece of the you're-not-too-old-and-it's-not-too-late puzzle. Creativity can stem from a tension, need, or conflict yearning to be satisfied—a path involving openness, curiosity, perseverance, and investment of attention (Csikszentmihalyi, 1996). In the second half of life, we can reflect on the paths we've taken and develop new invigorating, creative steps forward to reimagine and expand our pursuits. For example, Nobel Laureate Linus Pauling, Ph.D., reportedly published more scientific papers between ages 70 and 90 years old than earlier in his life. Benjamin Franklin invented bifocal lenses at age 78, and in his 80's Robert Frost presented his poem at the inauguration of John F. Kennedy. In her 90's, renowned anthropologist Dr. Jane Goodall, advocated world-wide for community-centered conservation and important issues for the well-being of our planet (Jane Goodall Institute, 2025).

How can we build a bridge of connection between life as we've known it and our next steps? How do we mediate between a pre-retirement identity and a retired identity? According to experts, it can be helpful to reimagine how we might use skills from the workplace in new ways, leaning into relationships, learning new competencies, and creating space for activities we may have thought about or wanted to try but not yet experimented with or achieved.

Transitioning to this new stage can be a time to rewire components of our lives as we think about ourselves and our roles in the world. It can be helpful to scope out what's ahead, considering not only finances and health but also anticipating what a daily schedule might look like, creating a reinvigorated identity and greater meaning as we build new life structures (Amabile, 2019).

Thus, we return to the title of this book, a title that I came up with two years ago before I reached today's chain link fence, "You're Not Too Old and It's Not Too Late." What do I believe as I write this today? What will be my next steps? And what are *your* next steps?

Together, in the following pages we will explore these questions.

Inspirations

Here are a few questions to help you awaken to new possibilities as you navigate this season of life, wherever you find yourself at midlife into older adulthood. You might find it helpful to record your ponderings in a notebook or journal or on your electronic device.

- What do you enjoy, do well, get lost in?
- What are you surprised by?
- What awakens your interests?
- When you get an idea or something strikes your interest, do you follow it or walk away from it?
- What do you love about your life and the state of the world?
- What do you dislike about your life and the state of the world?
- Do you look at issues and problems from various viewpoints and perspectives? How do you do this?
- How can you open to and express what moves you?
- When you wake up in the morning, do you have specific objectives and a structure that empowers you to use your time in meaningful ways?
- What have you always wanted to get to but have not yet explored?
- How do you make time for relaxation, quiet, reflection, and noticing each day?
- As you read these questions, what do you know for sure? What is your next right step? What openness would you like to create as you imagine and reimagine what's next?

This week I will consider what's next
with a more open perspective.
I will pause and reflect on what really matters to me.

CHAPTER 3

Rethinking Possibilities for
Ongoing Health at Any Age

Our beliefs and expectations about how we live as we grow older matter more than we may realize. Why does this matter? We may have more influence over our health and well-being than we think. This chapter offers transformative possibilities, inviting you to revisit your assumptions, shift your mindsets, and optimize your quality of life.

The mind and body are not separate entities. Mind, body, and spirit are interconnected within us, subtly and not-so-subtly influencing our health and wellbeing. Research reveals that our bodies are not necessarily the only limiting factor as we get older; rather, the mind has a huge influence on the body. Thus, our thoughts and ideas about perceived limitations can influence whether we are aging with greater well-being or not (Langer, 2009; Levy, 2009; Pangnini et al., 2019). Even subtle shifts in how we understand our health and performance can empower us toward greater vibrancy and fulfillment. In one study, people with a more positive self-concept about getting older lived 7.5 years longer than those with less positive stereotypes (Levy, Slade, Kunkel & Kasi, 2002).

What if we expand how we envision possibilities for living as healthfully as we can at midlife and beyond? In the landmark *counterclockwise* study, Harvard University psychologist Ellen Langer (2009) invited two groups of men to an experiment to turn back the clock. For just a week, one group lived and acted as though it were 20 years earlier. They turned off their modern electronics and were invited to be who they were in 1959, for example, talking about the politics and books of that period, sending photos of themselves, and writing a brief autobiography as though it were 20 years earlier. The second group simply reminisced about that era.

Remarkably, Langer's research found that the process of getting older is less fixed than most of us realize. The men in both groups showed marked improvements in overall well-being, including posture, weight, vision, joint flexibility, performance on intelligence tests, and other factors. While both groups showed positive outcomes in only a week, the men who lived and acted as if they were younger showed even greater improvement. The counterclockwise data makes the case that by shifting our thinking, language, and behaviors we can let go of arbitrary limits on health and well-being to live as healthfully as possible at any age.

Human life expectancy is now longer than at any point in recorded history, increasing by almost 40 years since the 1800's (Staudinger, 2020). Yet, in western culture, years of assumptions about aging influenced by science, media, and pervasive social pressures have reinforced stereotypes that older is *less than* younger. These negative stereotypes about aging typically begin long before we reach midlife when as young people we often accept limiting assumptions about aging without questioning their accuracy (Levy et al., 2002).

Today, these widespread, systemic biases continue to marginalize older people, pushing them to the sidelines of life (Gendron et al., 2016). Consider widely used terms, such as *frail, elderly, feeble, senile*, and words like *unattractive, downhill, negative, disabling, bad*, and *ugly*. This language emphasizes fears, reinforces negative stereotypes, and contributes to the questionable idea that declines in health and well-being are terrible and inevitable.

Alternatively, what if we shift toward intentionally and actively questioning the limiting beliefs with which western culture bombards us? Consider the fact that some cultures have greater reverence for elders than do other cultures. For example, the Japanese philosophy of *wabi-sabi* invites us to notice the *beauty* in age and nature's imperfections. The art of *wabi-sabi* treasures the cracks in a bowl and fills them with strands of gold and silver rather than discarding the bowl. This outlook, based on Buddhist teachings, views beauty through an alternate lens. *Wabi-sabi* speaks to the notion that what is natural is beautiful, including life's imperfections—calling us to embrace our flaws and the raw, natural, impermanent existence aspects of ourselves and others. This perspective on life empowers us to rethink our ideas about what is and expand toward a more generative mindset of *what could be.*

Ultimately, our lives involve a series of choices, whether intentional or unintentional. Our beliefs and expectations are products of our choices. One turning point can involve choices about living in authentic and real ways as we see ourselves with honesty, positivity, and self-compassion (Brown, 2010; Neff, 2011). We can face our vulnerabilities, while calling on our strengths and our courage, choosing to embrace who we are, imperfections and all. Exploring these options and decision points can offer greater introspection, new understandings, and an invitation to transform our beliefs about midlife and beyond from a mindset of inevitable, automatic decline toward greater empowerment, possibilities, mindful well-being, and a fuller life at any age.

Inspirations

This week consider the following self-inquiries to help you optimize your health and well-being in this season of your life:

- What do you know about living a healthy life?
- What negative stereotypes about aging have you been holding?
- How might your life be different if you softened to, accepted, and even prized the flaws and imperfections in your body and your life?
- How can you learn to make better choices about your health and well-being?
- What is your next right step toward rethinking possibilities for well-being and fulfillment?

***This week I will reconsider my thoughts
about growing older and awaken
to new visions of this season of my life and beyond.***

CHAPTER 4

The Resilience Factor -- Are You Getting Old or Growing Older?

A hardy red maple tree sits in my back yard. It stands vibrantly and serenely about 30 feet high—now. But it wasn't always that way. My mom and dad gave the young sapling to my young family about 25 years ago. Nobody would have predicted that this humble, crimson tree would survive the challenges it faced for it was planted in its burlap bag so that its roots grew tightly wrapped around its trunk. Yet, not only has it survived, but it has flourished, bringing resilience, beauty, shade, wisdom, and love into the lives of my family.

Sadly, my mom died last year. Like the tree, my mom withstood the many odds stacked against her in the 97 years of her long life. Even in her final days, like the maple tree, my mom shared profound lessons in resilience, beauty, wisdom, and love. Mom was still getting up and walking until just a few weeks before she died, when for the first time, she fell down and couldn't get back up. Until those moments, I believe my mom lived the definition of resilience, the ability to respond well to life's adversities (American Psychological Association, 2014). Throughout her long and meaningful life, she found a way to get back up each time life pushed her down.

No matter what age we are, we're all growing older every day. This is simply a fact of life. You might ask yourself "How can I live my best life? How can I flourish and thrive in *this* season of my life?"

In recent years, interest in adult developmental transitions has exploded with new descriptions including *the third act, second beginnings, second half of life*, and *renewment*. Not long ago, an informal conversation with a colleague resulted in brainstorming other monikers for this season of life, including *the wisdom years* and *wisdomhood* (B. Hurwitz, personal communication, March 14, 2025).

These revised concepts announce a renaissance for re-envisioning the process of growing older. In contrast to negatively biased stereotypes about hopelessly getting old with little influence on our thoughts and behaviors, the new paradigm conceptualizes the second half of life as a time of remarkable, perhaps unexpected, opportunities. A transformative shift in mindset invites openings for learning and deepening, emotional and spiritual development, increased freedoms, and engaging life in ways that amplify purpose, authenticity, and the wisdom acquired with experience.

Research by Laura Carstensen, Director of the Stanford University Center on Longevity, suggests a "positivity effect" as we grow older (Carstensen, 2006; Mather & Carstensen, 2005). Carstensen reports that older people tend to be happier and invest more personal resources in goals and activities they find emotionally meaningful. As people see their future timeframes as more limited, they are more likely to focus on feeling good in the present moment and tend to experience fewer negative emotions.

An important contributor to living as well as we can in any season of life is *resilience*, the capacity to adapt and respond to internal and external demands, transitions, and challenges (American Psychological Association, 2025). Resilience is about going forward, empowering ourselves at each stage of life to figure out what we can change, what we can't, and how we can live as fully and actively as possible.

Resilience skills help us get back up when we fall down, enabling us to adjust more effectively as we face stress, adversities, and difficult experiences. And here's very good news: resilient thoughts, skills, and actions can be learned, and anyone can develop them. There are thousands of resources available to help you cultivate and practice your resilience skills as well as those this book offers.

For each of us, the answers may differ, but some commonalities can point us toward living more resiliently at midlife and beyond. According to the *National Centenarian Awareness Project*, some of these commonalities include physical activity, a network of social contacts, a sense of humor, personal courage and strong will, a tendency toward optimism, and an ability to be adaptable in life (Adler, 1997-2017).

Inspirations

Midlife and beyond can be a time of transformative personal growth, new learning, and next steps, a blossoming toward strengthened resilience and new possibilities.

Here are a few strategies to help you flourish:

1 – **Embracing a perspective of optimism.** Change is part of life. Looking at experiences and events with an optimistic outlook can be empowering and heighten resilience (Snyder, Rand & Sigman, 2002).

You might experiment with visualizing, picturing in your mind's eye, what you *want*, rather than what you don't want. Imagine yourself taking the steps to achieve what you want in your desired situation. If an obstacle gets in your way, invite yourself to consider what other options might help you continue toward your objective. Meeting life's challenges with a positive perspective—glass half full rather than half empty—can bolster your sense of empowerment and your opportunities for resilience.

2 – **Reminding yourself to be flexible** – During challenging times, it's important to maintain perspective and invite yourself to be flexible. What can you alter and where do you have no control? When your plan A doesn't work, how about creating a plan B or plan C? Remember that life is not black-and-white. There is typically lots of ambiguity and gray area. Step back and gain perspective by looking at the bigger picture in order to re-focus and energize yourself. When feasible, are there other resources and people who could offer assistance in some way? What other options can you consider?

3 – Building connections with family, friends, and community. Speak less and listen more deeply. Ask good questions and pay attention to the responses of others. Listening quietly and attentively can improve and deepen your connections, helping you become more aware of what's happening with other people, enabling them to be heard, and potentially strengthening your relationships.

4 – **Taking care of your physical health.** Self-care, in various forms, continues to be important in each season of life. Listen to your body. How can you add more movement into your day? How can you become more physically active in a way that is healthy for you? Consider simple ways to add easy moments of movement into your day. For example, parking farther from your destination, walking the long route around the grocery store or at home, getting up to move for a few minutes during each hour of sitting (such as while reading, watching TV or working on your electronic device), taking a stretching or exercise class at the gym or online.

When you begin an exercise regime, remember to start slowly and gradually build toward your goal. Check in with your health care professional on a regular basis and as needed.

The resilience factor is profoundly important in life. On my own life journey, I continue to fall down and get back up in the ebb and flow of my grief, memories, and enduring love for my family. I find myself thankful for the profound gifts they have shared with me, including lessons on resilience, relationships, meaning, and love. Along with gratitude, I carry hope that the interconnected world that nurtures the brilliance of the red maple will continue to resiliently offer beauty, light, wisdom, and love for current generations, for the generations to come, and for the humanity, earth, and unfolding cosmos that connect us all.

This week I will intentionally move toward greater resilience in this season of my life—one step at a time.

CHAPTER 5

What's So Great about Positive Psychology and How Can It Help You Flourish at Midlife and Beyond?

Positive psychology has invigorated my life, reshaped my ideas about aging well, and inspired the direction of my work. Sometimes called the science of happiness, positivity, or flourishing, positive psychology came into view as a branch of psychology in the late 20th century although its roots began to emerge long before that time. Martin Seligman and Christopher Peterson have explained that positive psychology scientifically studies the factors that make life worth living (Peterson, 2008; Seligman, 2011). Understandings and applications from positive psychology can transform how we think about life's possibilities as individuals, organizations, communities, and nations. Many of the practices you find in this book are informed by understandings from the field of positive psychology.

In the past, psychology primarily focused on people's problems and how to fix them. The pathbreaking wave of the positive psychology movement is turning some of these perspectives upside down by instead studying happiness, flourishing, and well-being. As a result, transformative new understandings are shedding bright lights on the factors that make us resilient, more able to respond to and bounce back from life's challenges. Positive psychology asks: What makes a good life? How can we get the most out of life? How can we live with greater wellbeing, targeting our strengths and resources, rather than staying stuck in our weaknesses or deficits?

Psychology's roots evolved from experts who offered important ideas about becoming our best selves. The father of psychology, Sigmund Freud, understood love and work as two factors we need to live well (Erikson, 1968). Humanistic psychologist Abraham Maslow proposed a hierarchy of needs, suggesting that only after we meet our basic needs—biological, physical, safety, and connections—can we move toward self-actualization, becoming our fullest selves (Maslow, 1987). Psychologist Carl Rogers (1961) proposed that we can develop toward our best selves through genuine, accepting relationships that support our personal growth.

Then in 1998, as president of the American Psychological Association, Martin Seligman laid the groundwork for positive psychology, calling for an intensive focus on resilience, well-being, happiness, personal strengths, and flourishing. Seligman and his colleague Mihaly Csikszentmihalyi (2000) began assembling multi-dimensional research on the factors that contribute to flourishing and living happier, more meaningful lives. It's not just about us as individuals; these life-affirming benefits extend to our relationships and communities, empowering us to forge positive momentum beyond ourselves.

What can positive psychology offer you at midlife and the second half of life? This science of flourishing invites you to explore your fuller potential and build on your strengths, focusing more on what's *right* with you, rather than what's wrong with you. Positive psychology offers practical applications and clear steps to inspire you to transform your potential into action (Kellerman & Seligman, 2023; Niemiec, 2018; Seligman et al., 2005). Examples would be fostering gratitude, growth mindset, positive emotions, optimism, relationships, engagement and flow, meaning, purpose, leveraging your strengths, and working toward goals. You can learn about these practices and others in this book.

Blending these concepts with what you already know, challenging assumptions that no longer work for you, shifting your mindset, and building these skills can empower you toward greater wellbeing, life satisfaction, meaning, and happiness. The pathways are *not* a secret. You can learn these strategies and then choose to experiment with whatever might be a good fit in your own life, family, and communities.

Inspirations

Here are four practical applications to inspire greater well-being, happiness and possibilities in the days ahead:

1 - **Best Possible Self Activity** - Take a few moments to imagine yourself in the future. Set a time period, for example: three months, one year, or three years. Include all the relevant areas of your life, such as relationships, learning, play, spirituality, finances, home, work, and physical health (Dean, 1999-2005). Think about engaging your fullest potential as you visualize your best possible self in each area of your life. Imagine and write down the details. This activity can help you move from vague, fragmented thoughts to a clearer vision of your possibilities and actions (Kellerman & Seligman, 2023).

2 – **Three Good Things Activity** – Each day this week write down three things that went well for you. For each item, write about why you think it happened, what it means to you, or how you could have it happen again in the future (Achor, 2012; Seligman et al., 2005; Seligman, 2011). This practice can help you train your brain to notice life's positives. If you like the activity, you might continue it on a regular basis.

3 – **Generate More Kindness** -- Set a goal for yourself to do something kind for someone each day this week. Alternatively, positive psychologist Barbara Fredrickson, Ph.D. (2009), suggests planning to do five new kindness acts in a single day. She recommends targeting acts of kindness that can make a significant difference and require some effort from you. For example, you might invite a neighbor for a cup of tea and conversation or take a friend to their appointment. Kindness can help you feel better and make a positive difference to the people around you. You can build on this strategy by creating a kindness day on a regular basis.

4 - **Learn more about Positive Psychology, Flourishing and Potential**. Information about positive psychology, along with its concepts

and applications is abundantly available via books, podcasts, TED talks, articles, and other resources. You can refer to the references at the end of this book for more ideas.

> *This week I will try at least one new action to inspire greater well-being and possibilities in my life.*

CHAPTER 6

Awakening Meaning and Transformative Experiences in Your Life

As far back as I can remember, I've wanted to write a book. It had long seemed to me that creating a book was a meaningful way to share important ideas with others and leave something here after I am no longer in this lifetime. This book-writing goal seemed significant but improbable. Honestly, except for writing my master's thesis and doctoral research project, the two lengthy documents necessary to culminate my educational endeavors, I never managed to find space in my busy life to write the book I aspired toward. Other activities always got in the way, until a few years ago.

For many of us, our days are frequently measured in timelines and checklists. "It's Friday, and I made it through the week." "I need to shop for groceries, get a haircut, and do the laundry." Although we may need to accomplish these tasks, we may want to ask ourselves how important they are in the big picture, the overall context of our lives. How do we create space in our lives to pause and consider what is truly meaningful to us or even potentially transformative? Self-discovery questions, such as this one, speak to the heart of amplifying meaning, purpose, personal transformation, and serving the greater good.

Happiness can be seen as a product of meaning; in other words, finding meaning in life is a building block for happiness (Frankl, 1985). Each season of our lives can offer opportunities to reflect on our priorities, values, and experiences in our personal lives and perhaps in the larger context of existence. If we are motivated to do so, we can ask ourselves what engages the heart. What experiences bring us joy, fulfillment and meaning, and which ones simply fill up our time and habits of mind. Some experiences, whether in our own personal spheres or among the external circumstances we encounter, can be potentially transformative while others are quickly forgotten.

Research shows that seeking meaning and purpose can enhance our health and wellbeing, helping us flourish (Seligman, 2002). The essence of meaning is about how we make sense of life events, the process of seeking purpose in our lives. Meaning is derived when we reach *beyond* ourselves as single entities toward greater awareness of a larger context (Baumeister et al., 2013; Frankl, 1985; Wong, 2016). How we assign meaning and what we assign meaning to is unique to each of us, and there are myriad ways to invest ourselves in seeking and discovering meaning.

Perhaps you are motivated to discover greater meaning and potential in your life and the situations you encounter. Asking yourself open, thought-provoking, potentially transformative questions about the experience or event can help you uncover greater insight, understanding, and meaning. When studying peak transformative experiences, even difficult experiences can be transformative and imbued with greater personal meaning (Naor, 2016).

The search for meaning is *not* a once and done milestone. On some level, we are always in the practice of self-discovery; seeking meaning can be an evolving process that ebbs and flows in the wake of life's challenges, transitions, and events. Author and life coach, Diane Dreher (2008), writes that seeking our calling in life is a process of discovery that continues throughout our years, informed by our questions, conflicts, and important dreams. How are you called toward meaning-seeking and meaning-making? How can you take intentional steps toward what you find meaningful in this season of your life?

Inspirations

This week you might experiment with pausing and looking inside yourself and your experiences. Pay attention to your sense of self, the meanings you make in life, how you see the world around you, and your potential as an evolving, whole person. You might want to write down your thoughts and ideas as you experiment with these exercises.

Inspiration Exercise 1:

- Invite yourself to sit quietly. Notice your aliveness, perhaps quietly observing the flow of your breath, the sensations in your hands, or the feel of the ground below your feet.
- Tune into your inner wisdom. What is something that really matters to you in your precious life that you have not yet created time for?
- How can you include this meaningful objective in your life even for a few minutes each day or each week?
- What is your first step?

Inspiration Exercise 2:

- On one or more days during this week, reflect on a recent experience in your life that you found meaningful.
- Whether you've chosen an enjoyable experience, a challenging one, or some other kind of experience, what did you find meaningful about it?
- What did you learn about yourself or the situation via this experience, or what can you learn?
- How might you have changed or grown because of this experience?
- As you reflect on this experience, what meaningful insight or transformational opportunity do you want to take forward into your life?

This week I will reflect on what is meaningful to me and consider how I might include more of it in my life.

CHAPTER 7

What Can Mindfulness
Do For You?

In my own life, practicing mindful awareness has powerfully transformed how I am present with myself and how I relate to the world. As I navigate the gifts and challenges of daily life, practicing mindfulness helps me navigate my day-to-day with more calm and self-compassion, inner balance, and effectiveness.

Cultivating mindfulness can positively enrich our lives on many levels. Although mindfulness has ignited an explosion of interest and research in contemporary times, its basic practices date back over centuries. Today's research sheds light on the numerous benefits of mindfulness for resilience, well-being, physical and emotional health, learning, and dealing more effectively with life's stresses (Matta & Jacobsen, 2025; Goleman & Davidson, 2017).

The term *mindfulness* is thrown around a lot these days. Mindfulness is actually quite simple, inviting us to learn to observe things clearly just as they are. Of course, while this practice is quite simple, it's not always easy. Jon Kabat-Zinn (2012), who founded the highly respected Mindfulness-Based Stress Reduction Clinic (MBSR) at the University of Massachusetts Medical School, describes mindfulness as intentionally paying attention non-judgmentally in the present moment.

There are many ways to tap into mindfulness and practice it in our lives. Mindfulness does *not* have to take a lot of time. Rather, we can think about mindfulness like a muscle: the more we exercise it, the stronger our ability to experience mindful moments can become. From this perspective, we can strengthen our mindfulness muscles with practice as we learn to weave mindful moments into what we already do in our lives.

Mindfulness teaches us *how* to pay attention. This is significant. Throughout our lives, we're told to "pay attention," but how do we do that? How do we pay attention, and how can we get better at it? When we pay attention—one moment at a time—we can navigate the turbulence in our life in a more grounded way, with greater awareness, equanimity, and well-being.

One of the many potential benefits of mindfulness is self-compassion. According to psychologist Kristen Neff, mindfulness is an essential ingredient for self-compassion, that is, accepting and treating ourselves with kindness and an open heart. Practicing mindfulness can help us clarify our experiences with less judgement and a greater capacity to see things as they are (Neff, 2011; Shapiro et al., 2007).

Inspirations

Life is busy with much to do. Do you feel overwhelmed, worry more than you want to, respond to too many emails? Perhaps you're thinking, "I see that mindfulness can be helpful, but I don't have time for it. Why would I want to include mindfulness in my life?" I invite you to consider that mindfulness does not pull you away from life's responsibilities, but rather being mindful can help you cultivate greater attention, energy, and enjoyment.

Constantly rushing and worrying about all we have to do can activate the stress response, waking up the release of hormones including cortisol, preparing our bodies to fight or flee. When confronted with dangerous situations, our stress reactions are vital for enabling us to react quickly to keep ourselves safe. However, in many everyday life situations, this automatic response may not be so helpful. The stress response can cause our bodies and minds to tense up when we feel threatened but not in danger, for example, when we go to the dentist's office, in a social situation, anticipating a meeting, appointment or presentation, or simply waking up in the morning. Chronically high or low levels of cortisol may affect sleep, blood pressure, or the immune system (Cleveland Clinic, 2025).

Remarkably, simply pausing and noticing your breathing (or choosing a different focal point if noticing your breathing isn't comfortable for you) can calm and soothe your body, mind, and spirit, helping you shift from a busy mind to a more centered state of being. We're not talking about deep breathing or changing your breath in any way, just paying attention to the breath, or another anchor that you prefer, such as noticing your feet touching the ground or a sound in your environment.

There are many ways to engage with mindfulness, even for brief moments, as you do what you already do during the course of any day. For example, you can pause to take a mindful moment when you wake up at the start of the day, before taking a bit of food or as you glance out a window.

Here's a mindfulness exercise you might want to experiment with (Neff & Germer, 2018; Willard, 2016). As mentioned, if focusing on your breathing is not comfortable, you might choose an alternative focus:

- Tense your fists firmly for a few seconds. Then, just notice how you feel.
- Now, begin to pay attention more mindfully. Relax your hands. Rest them comfortably, perhaps on your lap, while you simply notice your next few breaths. How do you feel now? What thoughts, emotions, and sensations are you experiencing?
- Then, gently place your hands on your heart space and take a few breaths. You do *not* need to change anything about your breath; simply notice your breathing as it is right now. What thoughts, emotions, and sensations are you experiencing?
- Now quietly *watch* your breath as you inhale and exhale for a moment or two. Again, you do *not* need to change anything at all. Simply notice.

- Take a moment to reflect on your experiences. What did you notice?
- If you'd like to further consider your experience with this exercise or other mindfulness practices, you might want to write about them in your notebook, journal or electronic device.

Practicing mindfulness can help you experience greater balance in your life. Including just a few moments to pause mindfully each day—to settle down and focus on your breathing or other focal point—can offer the potential for greater calm, self-compassion, and wellbeing.

How can you include a few moments of mindfulness in your day-to-day?

If you already practice mindfulness, how can you strengthen your practice by adding a bit more?

This week I will remind myself to pause for a moment or two of mindfulness each day.

CHAPTER 8

Embracing the Potential to
Discover, Change, and Grow

Let's face it: change is part of life's journey whether we are happy about it or not. Many of us struggle with push and pull as we navigate the interplay between change and the status quo, especially as we walk through adulthood at midlife and then into later seasons of our lives. We're asked to learn something new or do something differently, and we may think to ourselves, "No way. I can't do this."

Sometimes, the call for change, discovery, or growth comes from within us. At other points in our lives, we may be awakened by the voices or actions of others, our work, environments, or communities. The changing realities and possibilities that life throws at us can offer entryways with opportunities for discoveries, learning, and transformation.

Renowned Stanford University psychologist Carol Dweck identifies characteristics of what she has termed the *growth mindset*, a belief that we can change, improve, and achieve through effort, experience, and willingness to learn from our mistakes as well as from our successes (2006; 2014). In contrast, a person with more of a *fixed mindset* tends to believe we're born with a certain amount of ability and that's just who we are, with little room for growth or change. According to Dweck, our mindset can impact every facet of our lives, including our relationships, work, family, and personal/professional achievements.

Consider the possibilities here. With a growth mindset comes the belief that you can get better at something because your capabilities can blossom, with perseverance, effort and practice. Developing your skills can be transformational, building momentum and motivation to stretch toward your desired goals. For example, maybe you want to learn to walk more steps each day, play golf, sing, or develop your leadership skills. With a fixed mindset, you may believe, "I'm no good at this, so why bother trying?" Alternatively, with a growth mindset, you may believe, "I can solve this. I can learn and practice to build this skill. With experience, I can get better. Let's get started!"

Inspirations

Your thoughts, words, and actions matter and can help you strengthen your potential. This week, pay attention to your self-talk. Here are some questions to help you shift toward a growth mindset:

- What do I say to myself about my capacities to learn, solve problems, and grow?
- What can I learn from this experience or situation?
- What possibilities might this experience offer?
- How can I grow, improve, or change as a result?
- How can I learn to do this more effectively?
- How can I gain the insights, knowledge, skills, or resources I need to do this?
- What's my plan of action?
- What's the next right step?

In addition to observing your self-talk, you might pay attention to how you interact with others. Do the messages you share with people tell them they are limited and stuck, or do you let people know you believe in them and their potential?

Finally, consider these questions to inspire your growth mindset and empower your potential:

- How do I view mistakes and changes—as problems, or as opportunities for learning, problem solving, and growth?
- If I have a fixed mindset, how can I shift toward a growth mindset?
- How can I develop my potential and help others build their potential?
- How do I think about the value of *practice* and how do I engage with practice to strengthen my learning and skill-building?
- How can I notice the positives about a learning and development process even if the outcome is not the desired one?'
- How can I learn more effectively from my experiences?

**This week I will pay attention to my self-talk
as I embrace my potential to learn, shift, and grow.**

CHAPTER 9

Living Life as a
Marathon, not a Sprint

As we mature, we may understand more profoundly that success in life is about much more than talent and getting things done quickly. Building on small wins, staying focused, and good old stick-to-itiveness can be turning points in the playbook of our lives. This steadfastness in persisting toward our goals even when we feel like giving up is called *grit*.

The term *grit* may trigger sensations of gravel or sand between your teeth or maybe a bold, courageous character in a novel or movie. However, psychosocial grit is so much more meaningful. Researcher Angela Duckworth (2016) defines grit as a combination of passion and perseverance, the empowering mixture for building fortitude and living life as a marathon, not a sprint. Grit can bolster the tenacity to persist toward long-term goals despite obstacles (Duckworth et al., 2007).

According to Duckworth and her colleagues, gritty people share four factors.

- **Interest:** When we enjoy what we're doing, we're more engaged and feel rewarded by our endeavors. Developing our interests and passions helps us deepen and sustain interest over the long term.
- **Practice:** Deliberate practice is a key to continuous improvement (Ericsson et al., 2007). Importantly, not all practice is the right stuff. Effective practice is strengthened with focused concentration, effort, repetition, and identifying steps for further improvement.

- **Purpose**: Contributing to our own interests while *also* offering benefits to others is a key ingredient of grit. For example, a restaurant server may either view their work as simply bringing food to people or see their work as an opportunity to make a positive difference in the quality of each customer's day.

- **Hope**: Hope involves noticing possibility, engaging our personal agency to motivate ourselves, and acting in ways to take positive steps toward our goals (Snyder, 1994). Hope also means recognizing that, regardless of the outcome, our experiences are opportunities to learn and grow. Gritty hope is action-oriented and can stimulate positive momentum that helps us stay in the game toward our goals and desired outcomes.

Inspirations

This week, consider a goal you'd like to achieve.

- Are you tackling your goal as a sprint or a marathon? If you're not satisfied with your progress, how can you engage your grittiness to move forward, even if you feel like giving up?

- Think about how you might power up one or more of the four grittiness components—interest, practice, purpose, and hope—to propel yourself toward your goal. For example, write in your notebook or journal about your interest and purpose, and then brainstorm some ideas about how you might solidify your practice to produce the results you desire.

- Talk with others about your goal and why it's important to you.

- How can you gain greater focus on your goal?

- How can you return to your focus when you encounter an obstacle or when you get distracted?

- How can you engage your hope as you persevere toward your goal? Who might you invite to cheer you on and support you when you falter?

- What are your next steps toward completing the marathon?

This week I will show up with the grit to steadfastly keep going toward my goal even when I feel like giving up.

CHAPTER 10

Reflecting on Your Story as You Navigate the Stream of Your Life

I like to think that our humanity flows through the rivers and streams of our lifetimes. To be human is to have a story that meanders, twisting and turning through the shallow waters and deep currents of our days. Our stories matter. As we experience the changes and transitions on our lifetime journeys, each of us is a work-in-progress with stories waiting to be told. Where have you been, where do you want to be, and where are you going in life? Consider that this *where* may not necessarily be geographical. Rather, *where* can be a metaphor, inviting you to reflect more intentionally on where you have traveled and hope to travel in the flowing stream of your life.

At any age, reflecting on the course of your life can contribute to personal insights and understandings (Staudinger, 2001). At midlife and beyond, one strength that tends to expand and gain greater meaning is the capacity to look back and gain perspective. Life's second half can be a time of boundless inner growth, possibilities, and meaningful contributions to our world. This journey is often led by growth, a calling toward self-actualization, exploring your uniqueness and your best self as you navigate toward full potential (Maslow, 1943; 1987).

Research indicates that writing your story can stimulate biological changes and may keep you healthier longer (Pennebaker & Smyth, 2016). Psychologists James Pennebaker and Joshua Smith offer some pragmatic suggestions for expressive writing, including trying to write for 15 minutes per day for a least three to four days in a row. There are many ways to write. Experimenting with what works best for you is a solid approach. Find a quiet place where you're not likely to be disturbed. Whether you write by hand, type on an electronic device, or dictate into a recorder, it's often easiest and most helpful to write simply for yourself, without concern about spelling or grammar. Keep in mind that you can choose to either throw away or keep what you write.

The insights you gain as you stand back and take stock, reviewing and sharing your stories, can help steer your choices and decisions toward greater awareness, clarity, inspiration, and satisfaction in the days to come (Cowan & Thal, 2015; Jung, 1971; Stewart & Vandewater, 1999). What are the stories within which your life has flowed and continues to travel?

Inspirations

This week, consider the lenses through which you view your life. While you cannot change your past, you can reframe your understandings in ways that offer greater acceptance, meaning and growth. Acknowledging and interpreting your past can help you learn from mistakes, navigate transitions and changes, be more open to the future, and build bridges toward greater meaning in your life.

Wherever you find yourself in the flowing stream of your life, offer yourself the time to reflect. This internal spaciousness can provide opportunities to wander on the journey of your mind—to ponder, interpret, and learn from your life's voyages and experiences. While your life may seem like a random collection of events, it's really all one story— *your* story—the narrative of your life.

Find a safe, peaceful space to sit quietly in the present moment. When you're ready, gently bring your attention to the stream of your life. If you find that you'd like to be more systematic in your life review process, jotting down your thoughts in a journal, notebook or electronic device can be a powerful strategy.

Consider these questions as you create a map of where you've been and where you are steering toward.

- What are some of the significant stories of my life?
- What important lessons have I learned?
- What do I wish I'd learned sooner?
- What do I wish I'd done that I haven't done (yet)?
- What mistakes have I made that are important to share with others?
- If I could live my life again, what would I do differently?
- What do I value most?
- As I look back, what has been my calling in life.
- Where am I called to explore further or create action steps?
- What do I want to learn more about?
- What are my hopes—for my life? my loved ones? my country? the world?
- How do I want to share my reflections, understandings, and wisdom with others?

This week I'll begin to reflect on my own story as I navigate the flowing stream of my life.

CHAPTER 11

Readiness to Create
Positive Personal Change

When you're considering a positive personal change in your life, how do you know when you're ready to get started? Do you dig in, persevere, or give up?

What personal change are you considering? Do you want to *(fill in the blank)*: manage your time more effectively, declutter your home, lose a few pounds, share more time with family or friends, exercise more regularly, start a new sport or hobby, learn to play a musical instrument, meditate daily, or something else?

Decades of research indicate that *readiness* for personal change is a key ingredient for success. Behavior change typically happens gradually as we shift from little or no awareness/interest in considering the change, followed by planning and taking specific actions (Zimmerman et al., 2000). By understanding this process, we can proceed more effectively and with less discomfort.

Researchers outline a 6-phase cycle that has revolutionized understandings about creating personal change. Knowing about and engaging in these phases can help us navigate our goals and increase our possibilities to achieve them (Prochaska et al., 1995):

Phase 1 - **Not yet thinking about it**. We have little or no awareness that the behavior is a concern or causes negative consequences. We have no intention to change or feel unable to change.

Phase 2 - **Beginning to think about it and weighing the possibility.** We are giving some consideration to the change. We may see positives about making the transition, are beginning to think about moving in that direction, but have no true intention to take action.

Phase 3 - **Planning, setting goals, and beginning small steps.** We are getting ready, laying the groundwork and preparing the way. We're developing specific plans to create action within the next month and may already be moving toward the change.

Phase 4 - **Taking active steps to make it happen.** We are actively moving toward the goal, changing behaviors and making choices to move forward. Coping with challenges, we are building momentum toward manifesting our chosen personal change.

Phase 5 - **Keeping up the momentum, persevering to maintain and sustain the change.** We've made the changes and achieved the goal for a significant period of time and actively intend to keep it up going forward.

Phase 6 - **The changes become a well-practiced, long-standing habit.** The new personal behavior is automatic, and returning to the old behavior no longer tempts us.

Inspirations

If you're thinking about a change, consider these questions to discern your level of readiness:

- What are the benefits of changing this behavior? How will your life be better or different?
- What are the negative consequences of continuing an unwanted behavior or of not beginning a new behavior you want to start, such as taking up a new hobby?
- How does this behavior, or lack of it, get in the way of your ability to achieve your goals in life or at work?
- How ready are you to commit to what it takes to create and sustain the change?

How's your self-efficacy? Self-efficacy is believing you have the capacity to do what you say you'll do. When you believe you are capable of succeeding, you're more likely to work toward and achieve your goals (Bandura, 1997). Strategies such as observing others as role models, visualizing yourself taking action and achieving success, and talking about your wins can inspire you toward positive changes.

If you feel ready to change, here are some questions to consider:

- Are your goals and plans realistic?
- How can you engage your growth mindset (See Chapter 8) and grit (See Chapter 9) to help you accomplish your goal?
- What supportive people and resources can you call on for encouragement or to help you hold yourself accountable?
- What obstacles might get in the way and what are your options to deal with them?
- How will you celebrate your successful milestones?

This week I will consider a positive change I want to make and anticipate how ready I am to create it.

CHAPTER 12

Nurturing Strengths, Youth, and a Legacy for Future Generations

In this complex world, how can you interact with young people in your life in meaningful ways? Today's children and teens are the next generations who will lead this world far beyond our own lifetimes. Whatever our role, whether we are parents, grandparents, teachers, mentors, professionals, neighbors, friends, or fill any other societal role, we can offer positive, valuable contributions to inspire future generations. Even one caring, supportive adult who notices a young person and their potential can have a positive impact on that person's life.

Positive psychologist, Lea Waters, an expert on the science of strength-based parenting, recommends intentionally focusing on what is *right* with ourselves and others, emphasizing strengths. This does not mean ignoring weaknesses, rather it's about being aware of strengths and learning to engage them in positive ways.

Essentially, identifying our strengths involves knowing our capabilities and having a vocabulary to describe them. Researchers have developed several systems to classify strengths. Perhaps the most influential and well researched is the VIA Classification of Strengths and Virtues (Peterson & Seligman, 2004), which identifies 24 character strengths common to humankind. These strengths are curiosity, creativity, judgement, kindness, perspective, leadership, perseverance, bravery, zest, honesty, social intelligence, fairness, forgiveness, teamwork, love, gratitude, love of learning, self-regulation, spirituality, humility, appreciation of beauty, prudence, hope, and humor (Niemiec, 2018).

You can begin identifying your own strengths by thinking about a time when you were functioning at your best. Recall the details (Niemiec, 2014). Consider what you did, how you felt, and the impact or outcomes. What strengths did you use in that situation? How did you feel when you were at your best? Now that you're more aware of your strengths, ask yourself how you can engage them in a current life situation or to meet a current challenge.

Inspirations

A caring, supportive adult who focuses on strengths can motivate young people to discover their strengths and abilities and galvanize their self-concept. As you interact with young people in your life, how can you help them reach toward their fullest potential? Here are a few ways to learn more about your own strengths and help young people gain greater awareness of theirs.

1 - To gain greater awareness of your strengths, you can take the free VIA Character Strengths Survey at https://www.viacharacter.org/.

2 - Write a positive note or text or call a child or teen you know. You might include the strengths you see in them and what positive impacts they have had on you or others (Niemiec, 2018; Waters, 2017). Be as specific as possible.

If feasible, plan a visit with the youngster, read the note personally, and give it to them. Pay attention to their reactions. Then, discuss your feelings and theirs together.

3 - When children or teens in your life are struggling with a challenge, how can you support their strength development?

For example, you could ask: "Which of your strengths can you use here?" Then, offer a strength that you have noticed in the youngster in another situation. Or you might ask, "When you used this strength before, how did you use it and how did it feel? How can you use the strength in *this* situation?"

***This week I will identify my own
strengths and consider how I can help
a young person focus on theirs.***

CHAPTER 13

Planting Seeds in the Garden of Well-Being: Mindful Adults, Mindful Kids

*"There are two mistakes one can make along
the road to truth...not going all the way, and not starting."*

- The Buddha

Life unfolds moment by moment. The last chapter explored strengths and a focus on noticing what's *right* with youth in our lives. How can we help them and ourselves awaken to a more balanced way to experience moments in life?

Being a teacher, parent, and grandparent has shown me how sharing mindfulness with children and teens is similar to planting seeds in a garden (Berns-Zare, 2018). As Jon Kabat-Zinn reminds us, mindfulness is simply paying attention purposefully in the present moment (2012).

Pause, breathe, notice, return. These simple actions that can be gently practiced with intention and integrated into everyday life, helping us cultivate quiet interiority, internal spaciousness, and well-being.

How do *you* want to be present as you engage with young people?

Whatever your role in the lives of young people, nurturing mindfulness can begin with you and your own practices, your own way of being in the world. There are many ways to practice mindfulness, and this does *not* have to involve the stereotypical thirty minutes of silence sitting still on the floor. Mindfulness practices vary as our lives unfold, and the skills can be adapted for anyone from young children to adults in any season of life.

Strong evidence links mindfulness with positive emotions, enhanced life satisfaction, compassion, and overall wellbeing. Mindfulness practices can help people experience greater balance and calm, reducing risk for illness, and bolstering physical and emotional health (Goleman & Davidson, 2017; Willard, 2016). Psychologist Lea Waters (2017) points to the benefits of mindful parenting. Gains can include improved parenting in the moment, modeling effective ways to deal with relational conflicts and stressful situations. Mindful adults can coach youth to grow toward greater mindfulness in their lives.

It's hard to share mindfulness with kids if we haven't experienced it ourselves. Planting the seeds of mindfulness in our own lives, engaging in mindfulness practices, and modeling mindful awareness for young folks can inspire them to become interested and motivated to try it themselves. Just one breath with awareness and gentle attention offers the potential to transform any moment or any situation.

I enjoy spending peaceful time with my grandchildren doing ordinary things like walking at the park, digging in the garden, sitting under a tree to play a game, or watching a bird flying by. Yet, recently when my boisterous granddaughter was struggling with something I had asked her to do, my initial impulse was frustration. But rather than responding impulsively, I intentionally paused for a mindful inhale and exhale. That deliberate breath awareness created a brief, but meaningful intermission. Notably, just that simple pause to notice my breath empowered me so that I could respond more calmly, thoughtfully, and patiently, rather than quickly and harshly.

Inspirations

Here are a few approaches to consider this week as you cultivate mindfulness in the garden of your life.

1 - S.T.O.P. -- This easy acronym is a reminder to plant the seeds of mindful moments in your daily life (Goldstein, 2013).

- **S**top
- **T**ake a breath
- **O**bserve (notice feelings, thoughts, sensations without judgement)
- **P**roceed

STOP can be practiced in the context of ordinary activities, such as morning awakening, brushing teeth, walking to the kitchen for breakfast, during a break, before a meal, in bed at night.

2 - 3 R's Practice: Rest, Recognize, Return – This simple practice may help when your mind wanders (Willard, 2018).

- **REST** your awareness – You can use an "anchor" to help you focus your attention (Shonin, et al., 2015). For example: Noticing the flow of your in-breaths and out-breaths; silently repeating a brief sentence or mantra, such as *I am breathing in. I am breathing out." or* focusing on a word, such as peace, calm, love, quiet.
- **RECOGNIZE** when (and where) your mind and thoughts wander.
- **RETURN** to your anchor when you notice your attention wandering. Repeat this process as many times as needed.

3 - Plant seeds to nurture your garden of well-being – Consider these self-inquiries. You might want to take some notes about your thoughts and ideas.

- How can you incorporate a few moments of mindfulness in your day?
- If you already practice mindfulness, how can you add a bit more?
- How can you share moments of mindfulness with the youth in your life?

4 – Inspiring young people to develop more mindful awareness
In your busy day-to-day, you and the children in your life may forget

to pause. Notice opportunities to inspire youth as you introduce and model seeds of mindfulness. For example:

- Model mindful moments as you introduce the practice to the youth in your life - Let children see you pause and breathe mindfully when you are upset or before you respond impulsively in a challenging situation. Explain to them what you are doing and how you find it helpful. Invite them to try it with you.

- Occasionally, find a quiet space for brief moments with a youngster. You might read a book together, share a conversation, express love and gratitude, take a walk, or say a prayer together.

- Sometimes, a child may prefer to sit quietly by themselves for a few moments. You might simply sit quietly near them or walk away and give them a bit of space. Pay attention to what feels comfortable for the child and honor their needs.

This week I will cultivate more moments of mindfulness in the garden of my life.

CHAPTER 14

Strong Life Purpose and Your Quality of Life

Having a sense of purpose in any season of life may be one of the most potent components of resilience and wellbeing. What gives you a sense of active engagement and makes your life feel valuable and worth living? When was the last time you paused to consider what is truly meaningful to you?

Whether you are actively working in or outside your home, anticipating retirement, or retired, how do you think about your life currently and imagine it going forward? A growing number of studies shows connections between a sense of purpose, health benefits, longevity, and overall quality of life (Alumujiang, et al., 2019; Cohen et al., 2016; Hill & Turiano, 2014; Martela et al., 2024). While it's important to realize that correlation is *not* causation, accumulating evidence supports the notion that purpose in life is associated with length and quality of life.

With people transitioning to retirement from work in record numbers, the pursuit of purpose has become a topic of increasingly broad and compelling relevance. Intentionally exploring purpose and meaning can open doors to cultivate well-being as you navigate the challenges and opportunities in the second half of life. Perhaps these findings suggest a noteworthy mindset shift from a *retirement of leisure* toward a *retirement of meaning and purpose.*

Leaders in positive psychology explain meaning and purpose as cornerstones of happiness, flow, optimal experience, and a well-lived life (Csikszentmihalyi, 1990; Fredrickson, 2009; Seligman, 2011). Stanford University psychologist William Damon and his colleagues, Menon and Bronk (2003), define *purpose* as a steady intention to achieve something meaningful to ourselves and significant to the world beyond the self. Their definition of purpose includes three components:

1. Purpose is *more* than simple day-to-day objectives, such as getting dinner on the table or driving to work. Rather, it's about having goals and a sense of direction.
2. Purpose involves stretching or reaching out in some way beyond ourselves.
3. Purpose often includes progress, achievement, or completion.

Purpose invites you to define goals and ideals that are personally and deeply meaningful, calling you to reach beyond yourself in a way that progressively defines your identity. Purpose does not have specific definitions or boundaries. Whether you experience a sense of purpose as, for example, a receptionist, parent, grandparent, gardener, carpenter, teacher, caregiver, musician, volunteer, or activist does not matter. It is having a sense of purpose that does matter. Purpose—whether large or small, whether you reach your objective or continue to strive for it—can transform your life in very important ways that can transform your physical and mental health and overall well-being.

Inspirations

What gives you a sense of purpose in your life? Do you deliberately engage in activities you find meaningful and that energize you? *You* are ultimately responsible for asking the questions and searching for the answers to what is engaging, meaningful and relevant for you in your life, work, and community. Thinking intentionally about what you care about can help you clarify your sense of purpose and how you live your life.

Here's an activity to help you tap into what brings you feelings of purpose and meaning (adapted from Niemiec, 2018).

1 – Consider these questions: What matters *most* to me? What are my dreams, goals, and challenges? What have I learned about what's truly important? What are my values and character strengths? How am I making a difference in the world, and how would I like to make a difference?

2 –As you ponder these questions and others that might occur to you, imagine how you'd *like* your life described to the next generation. Write a short summary, story, or bullet-points telling your story, as you'd like it to be told, in as much detail as you'd like.

3 - Set the summary aside for a few days and then re-read it. What stands out to you about the story? What values and strengths do you notice in your story? What similarities and differences do you notice between the story you'd like to tell and your actual life? How does the story you wrote fit with what is truly meaningful to you?

4 – Take some time to reflect. Consider talking with others you trust or respect about your story and what you find meaningful.

5 – Are there any shifts you want to make in your life? If so, what are you considering? How will your priorities shift if you choose to pursue one or more of your meaningful objectives? What would it require if you chose to work toward this goal?

6 – What action step(s) are you ready to take?

This week I will invite myself to notice what brings me a sense of purpose and meaning and consider how I can add greater purpose to my life.

CHAPTER 15

Practicing Self-Care in the
Big Picture of Your Life

As you navigate adventures, challenges, and transformative possibilities of your current life and anticipate the years ahead, how do you envision your relationship with your own self-care? Do you have, or want to have, intentional goals for how you care for your body, mind, and spirit, your holistic well-being? What is your long-game plan for your self-care, well-being, and how you might approach living your best life now and, in the years, to come?

The question "How shall I take care of myself" is not a new or unique inquiry. In the first century, renowned Jewish sage Rabbi Hillel asked, *"If I am not for myself, who will be for me? If I am only for myself, what am I? If not now, when?"* (Herford, 1962). Rabbi Hillel's questions awakened life adventurers then and now to pay attention to personal callings and responsibilities—to compassionately care for and harvest the bounty of our own lives, as we also compassionately engage with the world around us.

In the big picture journey of your life, where are *you*? Consider the idea that perhaps this is not a geographical question, but rather an invitation to reimagine the big picture of your life as you look into yourself as a whole being.

As we grow in maturity and face the variety of transitions life serves us—whether in young adulthood, midlife, or elderhood—our relationship to self-care evolves and changes. Along with our individual health and wellness, we may notice inner stirrings of the self, along with new understandings, meanings and experiences.

Practicing self-care is associated with greater wellbeing and there are many ways to take care of yourself (Posluns & Gall, 2020). Self-care is not about perfection. It's much more about embracing our wellbeing with intention and awareness in ways that fit our life situations, our capacities, interests, and needs, and our level of motivation to empower ourselves to live better longer. Of course, *better* has different meanings for each of us. But many of us may desire to learn about ways to rethink how we approach our self-care, ways we can be proactive, rather than reactive. We may want to revise how we prioritize the care and sustenance of mind, body, and spirit with healthy choices and behaviors (Attia, 2023).

Inspirations

These topics are not once and done questions. They can be jumping-off points for a lifetime of self-exploration and seeking better ways to stay vital and live the best life you can. As you delve into these questions, consider talking with a partner or friend to share thoughts, stories, and strategies. You may also find it beneficial to reach out to a helping professional to delve into options.

Here are a few inquiries you may want to explore:

- What does the question *"If I am not for myself, who will be for me?"* bring to mind for me in this season of my life ?
- How has my self-care changed over time?
- What is my current relationship with self-care?
- Who do I think of as a positive role model for self-care?
- When do I feel younger? When do I feel older? How does my self-care reflect these differences?
- If I were to live "better," what might that mean for me?
- What habits in my life serve my self-care well, and what habits might I want to change, let go of, or begin?
- How can I befriend my body, mind, and spirit in new ways?

- What intentional actions can I take to improve my self-care?
- How will I hold myself accountable for this action?

***This week I will explore my relationship
with self-care at this time in my life.***

If not now, when?

CHAPTER 16

Cultivating Resilience and Positive Emotions amid Life's Ups and Downs

Our lives are complex and nuanced. Each day our choices affect our own lives and can influence those around us. As we accumulate birthdays in whatever decade of our lives we find ourselves, we confront uncertainties and opportunities. How do we discern where to focus our attention, thoughts, hearts, energies, and actions? How may we live the best lives we can as we navigate joys and adversities along our path?

This book speaks from a voice of resilience, vitality, and making the most of our ever-changing lifetimes. At times, this positivity can seem quite dissonant with the turbulence, transitions, and tragedies that life serves up. And yet, as humans, we are endowed with a drive to grow toward our full potential (Maslow, 1943). As we travel through midlife and beyond, life's ups and downs offer a multitude of opportunities for growth, discoveries, and meaning. With the personal resources and wisdom accumulated throughout our lifetime, each of us is called to respond to whatever life serves up as we live, work, and prepare the world for the next generation.

Viewing our struggles from a vantage point of positivity can strengthen our resilience, enabling us to acknowledge the wholeness of our experience: the darkness and also the light, the negative and also the positive, the sadness and the joy. Even when we're unable to recognize the sunlight behind the clouds, we are reminded that it's always there, just as the oxygen in the air is not visible, but we can notice it as our lungs inflate like wings with each breath.

Pleasant emotions offer much more than merely good feelings in the moment. They can help us experience greater well-being, cope more effectively, and even flourish during uncertain and difficult times (Bonanno & Keltner, 1997; Fredrickson et al., 2003). During stressful experiences, positive emotions can expand our thinking and attention, sparking new learning, ideas, and creativity. This *broadening* strengthens our emotional, social, physical, and cognitive reserves so we are more able to take positive actions as we adapt to circumstances in which we find ourselves (Fredrickson, 2004, 2009; Layous & Lyubimirsky, 2014).

How can we sustain ourselves and thrive amid life's struggles, adversities, and obstacles? Research shows that even during difficult times, tapping into our capacity to notice and experience positive emotions can help us create a healthier, more resilient life. Positive emotions, such as love, interest, gratitude, enjoyment, happiness, hope, optimism, and awe can empower us to expand our awareness, recognize that we are not alone, and harness our capacity to live the best lives we can as we respond to life's challenges.

According to University of North Carolina social psychologist, Barbara Fredrickson, it's important to seek a balance between positive and negative emotions (2009, 2020). Although negative emotions naturally arise in difficult situations, generating positive emotions helps build resilience, our ability to bounce back from life's challenges.

Importantly, cultivating positive emotions and a positive outlook does *not* mean that we never experience negative feelings, such as loneliness, sadness, frustration, or anger. Positive emotions are *not* something we can grab and hold onto tightly; emotions come and go in the breezes and storms of our days. Yet, we can strengthen our experiences of positive emotions while also acknowledging their fragility and impermanence. As such, shining a light on resilience and positivity isn't about turning away from life's challenges or forcing happy feelings when they are inappropriate to the situation. Many of us know from our own experience that forcing ourselves to feel happy when we don't may cause us to feel even worse. Instead, employing positive emotions while also recognizing our challenges can strengthen us as we ride the ups and downs of life, helping us notice slivers of sunlight when the journey seems dark and difficult.

One positive emotion that can help us face our challenges is hope, which can empower us to acknowledge our fear that the worst may happen, while yearning for and seeking something more (Fredrickson, 2009; 2020; Smith & Lazarus, 1991; Snyder, 1994). With hope, we can learn to grasp the wholeness of our experience – the positive and the negative feelings -- as we adapt to the ever-evolving demands of our lives.

Resilience and positive emotions can be major contributors to well-being at any stage of life. As you navigate life's inevitable twists and turns, more intentionally noticing and generating positive emotions can help you cope with life's turbulence and transitions, enhancing your ability to thrive.

Inspirations

This week, invite yourself to try one or more of these approaches to inspire your experience of positive emotions.

1 - What positive emotions are in your life toolbox? Consider a current challenge in your life. What has the whole of that experience been like for you? How could you leverage a positive emotion to help you reframe or respond to the situation with perhaps a glimmer of greater resilience?

2 – Do something that helps you generate a positive emotion. Examples of positive emotions include enjoyment, satisfaction, contentment, thankfulness, amusement, enthusiasm, happiness, affection, love, interest, confidence, hope, optimism, and awe. Create an opportunity to experience this positive emotion, perhaps with a social visit or phone call, a good deed, moving your body more actively, or simply noticing a good moment in your day.

3 – Each day this week take a moment to pause, notice, and write down a positive experience. It's ok to start with small steps. Even the briefest experience can offer at least a fleeting moment of positive emotion.

4 - Consider a time in your life when you felt bombarded by a challenge, and then found your way forward. What experiences, actions, and positive emotions helped you venture from darkness toward light?

5 - Think about someone in your own life or in popular culture who is a role model for resilience. How has this person responded to a tough situation, loss, or tragedy? What can you learn from this person to bring into your own life?

***This week I will intentionally add more
moments of positive emotions into my life.***

CHAPTER 17

Simply Noticing
Moments in Your Life

How are you present in the day-to-day of your precious life?

Where are you right now?

What are you noticing in this very moment?

Without pausing to intentionally notice life's moments, we are not as self-aware, balanced, or effective as we might be. When we are constantly busy, without occasional intermissions to notice the moments of our lives, it's as if we've turned off our internal cellular phone. There's lots of data coming in, but we can't hear the messages. To gain access to the information, we need to pause, notice the phone is off, and activate it. If we don't intermittently pause to notice our internal awareness, we may be oblivious to life's messages and meanings, whether simple or complex. We may not notice our own internal knowings or the realities of the people in our lives, the organizations in which we work or volunteer, and the world in which we live.

Mindfulness is really just about noticing the present moment. It's so simple that all we need to do is pause and pay gentle attention. And what is noticing? Noticing is simply focusing our attention, empowering ourselves to get out of autopilot, and to become more aware of our internal process without being blown away as frequently by the winds of life. Mindful leadership author, Maria Gonzalez (2012) writes that mindfulness principles can be woven into every aspect of our personal and professional lives, helping us make wiser decisions and increase our effectiveness.

Anyone can notice. Pausing to notice is a skill we can learn and exercise. Rather than being an all-or-nothing capability, noticing can be practiced step-by-step, moment-by-moment, like learning to read, cook, or drive a car. And noticing is available to all of us. It's *not* just for the old or the young, or the leader or the worker, or the believers or the non-believers. Noticing can be cultivated by *anyone.*

Even brief daily mindful pauses can transform our lives and our well-being at deep levels. These learnable practices support holistic well-being of the brain, spirit, and body (Goleman & Davidson, 2017; Siegel, 2011). Mindful attention can inspire us as individuals and also as part of the human community, companion travelers in our workplaces, organizations, and the world in which we live (Salzberg, 2014).

Not long ago, I tried a *noticing experiment (Berns-Zare, 2020a)*. Each day for a week I paused three times during the day for less than a minute to *just notice.* I set the calendar on my phone to remind me to pause, take a breath, and simply notice where I was and what I was experiencing. The results from my experiment were simple yet remarkable. These few seconds several times daily helped me feel just a bit calmer and gain greater clarity. I found that after a few days of this practice I began to pause and notice at other points through the day.

Inspirations

At its essence, mindfulness is *simply paying attention*. There are countless ways to gently pause and pay attention right here, right now. Here are 20 inspirational ideas to help you practice this simple, powerful way to transform the moments of your life.

1. Pause between bites of food.
2. Listen carefully with no agenda.
3. For just a few breaths, observe that you are breathing: in breath, out breath.

4. Pay attention to what you're doing right now.

5. Notice your surroundings.

6. Pay attention as you whisper a short blessing, prayer, or favorite quote.

7. Stop for a moment and be present quietly.

8. Gently move your body as you are able and notice how you feel.

9. Read an inspiring poem.

10. Turn off your electronic device(s) for an hour.

11. Sing a song in the shower—just for fun, no judgement.

12. Observe the sunrise, sunset, or moon shining at night.

13. Notice the birds singing.

14. Listen to music.

15. Notice something you enjoy in your surroundings.

16. Write a personal note of gratitude to someone that you appreciate.

17. Pause while you brush your teeth or wash your hands.

18. Notice when you are smiling and how it feels.

19. Play with a child or a pet.

20. Meditate.

What other ways to simply notice would you like to add to this list?

***Each day this week I will experiment with gently
noticing moments in my life,
knowing that even the briefest moments matter.***

CHAPTER 18

Intergenerational Relationships Can Be a Winning Formula for Young, Old and In-Between

Recently, a young adult friend, several decades my junior, celebrated a milestone birthday. We'd been professional acquaintances who realized we had compelling mutual interests and commonalities. During a recent conversation, she asked a powerful question about my life in the decade of my 30s. This discussion provoked important self-reflection and understanding about myself during that decade, and, I suspect, also provoked greater insight for her. She and I often learn from each other, exploring our shared interests and differences in our experiences, understandings, and the day-to-day of our lives.

I feel fortunate to have benefited from several meaningful intergenerational relationships, which began at different stages of my life, from my teens to the present. Sometimes, I have been the elder in the friendship, and at other times, I've been the junior member of the pair. The benefits of meaningful connections between young and old are often not recognized.

Yet, meaningful intergenerational interactions—family, friend, and social relationships between people of different generations—can enrich the lives of all involved, e.g., sharing wisdom learned via life's experiences and building skills to strengthen social and emotional intelligences.

These valuable connections can be a win-win for participants and are an overlooked resource in the United States.

Over 75 years ago, the landmark Harvard Longitudinal Study of Adult Development began studying more than 700 men, later expanding to include women. Remarkably, this research has shown over time that adults who engage in meaningful relationships with younger generations are more likely to feel happier, less stressed, and more optimistic than others without these relationships (Newberry, 2023; Waldinger, 2015, 2022).

And what about the benefits for young people? Psychologist Urie Bronfenbrenner, a founder of the U.S. Head Start preschool program, is quoted as saying, "Every child needs at least one adult who is irrationally crazy about him or her" (Stanford Center on Longevity, 2016, p. 7). Research at the Stanford University Center on Longevity reveals three important factors that can nourish young people's capacities for resilience and flourishing: (1) good emotional wellbeing and mental health cultivated by social interactions, support, and learning from others who possess these skills; (2) a sense of purpose; and (3) meaningful, caring social connections to help learn fundamental skills that can help them strengthen adaptive functioning and development.

Research findings illustrate the positive benefits of teaming up young and old in meaningful, purposeful relationships. (Kessler & Staudinger, 2007; Stanford Center on Longevity, 2016). Robust and caring relationships are linked to greater resilience and wellbeing for participants at all ages and stages of life. There are many skills and practices that cannot be gained in books, social media, or the internet, but that can be vigorously boosted via intergenerational relationships. And while enriching the lives of mature adults, purposeful intergenerational interactions can contribute to the wellbeing and life skill development of forthcoming generations, the future of our world.

In this tumultuous 21st century, there has never been a more important time to think about the mutual benefits of intergenerational relationships. You might be surprised to know that since 2015, the United States is home to more people over age 60 than under age 18 (Friedman, 2021). The population of adults over the age of 60 is a rich and untapped resource. Today's American populace is not simply living longer. Many are healthier cognitively, physically, and emotionally than previous generations. And plenty of mature adults are highly motivated by a desire to give back to others.

In his groundbreaking model of human psychological development, Erik Erikson was the first to describe the unfolding of *generativity* at midlife and beyond (Erikson, 1963; Malone et al., 2016). Many midlife and older adults are well-suited to mentor younger people, sharing knowledge, wisdom, and ideas, such as navigating the challenges of daily life, problem solving, critical thinking, social skills, decision-making, and perspective-taking. According to Harvard professor Arthur Brooks (2022), while young adults may solve problems more swiftly, older adults tend to be wiser about what problems are worth solving.

How can we promote healthy relationships between generations? Perhaps the first step is to simply be aware of the benefits of intergenerational interactions and then seek out opportunities to engage in healthy and meaningful ways with people not only of our own age but also those younger and older. Robert Waldinger, director of the Harvard Longevity Study, encourages us to build our "social fitness" (2022). Relationships don't just happen. We need to seek them out, tend to them, and take care of them.

Inspirations

Relationships across ages, interactions with friends, family, acquaintances, and communities can strengthen your wellbeing and happiness. Healthy, meaningful relationships between young and old can be mutually beneficial, helping each generation blossom toward their purpose and potential. How can *you* connect across generations? Do you take the initiative to safely reach out to others beyond your own age group?

In your own life and community, consider how you might get more involved in interactions or service with youth or young adults. Dr.

Waldinger suggests getting more comfortable simply starting up casual interactions with others during your day (2022). For example, pausing to say hello or having a brief conversation with someone you meet when you're taking a walk, shopping, sharing a meal, or connecting with others around shared interests. You might want to establish some routines that increase opportunities to engage with others intergenerationally, as well as in your own age group. To engage with others of different ages, you might seek opportunities to volunteer through local organizations, such as a local teen center, township office, senior center, religious organization, scouting, school programs, tutoring at a local library or school, or getting involved in special programs (Berns-Zare, 2025).

Engaging in intergenerational relationships can be enriching and transformative for young and old across generations. How might *you* help to make a positive difference?

This week I will consider the potential benefits of intergenerational relationships.

Is there a way I can engage in one or more positive interactions?

CHAPTER 19

Savoring and Enjoying
the Positive Moments

How often do you pause to enjoy a moment of pleasure in your life?

When something *good* happens, do you pay attention to the occurrence or experience? How often do you *not* notice positives when they're right in front of you? What do you say to yourself when you *do* notice or enjoy a positive experience?

Choosing to direct your attention to appreciate positive moments in your life that might otherwise be ignored or forgotten is termed *savoring*. The mental habit of savoring invites you to intentionally focus on positives, potentially expanding the enjoyment and appreciation you may draw from these experiences (Fredrickson, 2009; Stone & Parks, 2018).

Taking momentary pleasure in life's positive occurrences can help you experience greater happiness and well-being (Jose et al., 2012). Savoring is something kids and any of us can do. The benefits of this phenomenon seem to have no age limits. Research on older adults indicates that savoring boosts positive emotions, as well as resilience, the capacity to rebound from life's adversities (Smith & Hollinger-Smith, 2014; Wilson & Sakolofske, 2018).

Savoring involves intentionally choosing where to focus your attention in *this* moment. This kind of attention is *not* about analyzing or defining the experience but rather momentarily, mindfully appreciating any aspect of the experience that calls to you. It is about taking in the good, the pleasant experience, or special moment. For example:

- noticing the sensory sensations of something you enjoy—the visual, smell, sound, taste, or touch;
- intentionally recalling a positive moment from an earlier time;
- relishing a positive experience with another person as it's occurring;
- discussing the pleasure of a past or anticipated experience;
- pausing to feel or express a moment of gratitude or thankfulness;
- remembering something that we are hopeful about, proud of, or that makes us laugh.

Inspirations

This week how can you savor the positives in your life? You can experiment with the practice of savoring by slowing down for a moment or longer, paying attention, and appreciating one or more positive experiences in your life. Here's a savoring practice you can try:

1. One or more times each day (whatever timing works for you), quiet your mind for a moment and gently remind yourself to simply notice something positive about the present moment. Another option is to think about a positive occurrence that happened at a different point in time.
2. Choose one positive experience to appreciate. Just notice it. Perhaps consider what you enjoy about it.
3. How do you feel as you savor this experience?
4. When you're ready, simply go on with your day.

***This week I will give myself a moment or more
each day to pause and savor a positive experience.***

CHAPTER 20

Inspirations for Joy, Meaning, and Relationships

Each day, we make thousands of decisions and choices from our unique viewpoints that inform our reality as we experience it. As we navigate the second half of life, how can we create and notice experiences that inspire greater joy, meaning, and relationship? Whatever decade of life we find ourselves in, we have the choice to purposefully notice where we've been, where we're going, and perhaps most important, where we are right now in the present moment. Our observations and how we interpret them are windows that actively inform and transform how we experience our lives and the world around us.

The Dalai Lama, head monk of Tibetan Buddhism, reminds us that happiness grows from our actions (2017). And scientific research indicates that while good genes are welcome, our behaviors and choices can matter quite a lot.

Adult development research from the Harvard Study of Adult Development offers important insights on adult development and aging (Vaillant 2003; Waldinger, 2015, 2004).

Highlights from the Harvard study:

- Good relationships and social support, such as friends, family, volunteering, and social groups, positively benefit health and well-being.

- It's the quality of relationships, *not* the number of relationships, that makes the difference.
- Awareness that life is short makes people happier. Knowing that time is limited encourages people to prioritize well-being as important.
- Education and life-long learning are good for health, wellness, and longevity.
- Four actions that contribute mightily toward a happy retirement are: replacing work relationships with other social networks; re-discovering the act of playing; engaging in creative activities; and continuing to learn.

Positive relationships are one of the cornerstones of a fulfilling life. Christopher Peterson, (2006) an influential researcher in the field of positive psychology, is known for his visionary work on the factors that promote human potential and a life well-lived. Peterson frequently declared that "other people matter." Relationships, even brief positive moments of connection, contribute to emotional and physical health, well-being, and the way we experience our lives. Relationships are central to the components of flourishing that feed into wellbeing, known as PERMA (**P**ositive emotions, **E**ngagement (flow), positive **R**elationships, **M**eaning, and **A**ccomplishments) proposed by Peterson's pioneering colleague, Martin Seligman (2011).

Research shows that love and relationships can actually change the body's chemistry (Fredrickson, 2013). In other words, humans are hard-wired for connectedness and oneness. *Positivity resonance,* a term coined by Fredrickson, explains that when you share positive emotions with another person—even momentarily—there is a synchrony between your biochemistries and behaviors, which can result in mutual connection and investment in each other's well-being (2013). She calls these small positive interactions *micro-moments of connection.* Dr. Fredrickson suggests that the secret to building more positivity is to increase pleasant moments over time (Fredrickson, 2009).

Inspirations

There are many ways to create more joy, meaning, and relationships in your life. Here are some ideas to help inspire more moments of joy, meaning, and relationships.

1 – **Pausing for even fleeting moments of connection.** Take a moment to say hello to people as you go through your day—the cashier at the grocery store, the mail carrier, your neighbor, colleague or co-worker. Ask how that person is and actually listen to their response.

2 - **Relying on and helping other people.** Build social connections. Hang out with friends and family. Foster relationships in which you can count on other people, and they can count on you. Become involved in groups, organizations, and communities, whether in-person or virtually. For example, join a spiritual group, try an activity at the community center, take a class, or volunteer at a public library or an animal shelter.

3 – **Creating a greater sense of purpose, calling, and commitment.** Let a meaningful or challenging event stimulate you to think about what is truly important to you. Sit quietly and pay attention to what your inner knowing is saying. When you have a few free moments, reflect on or journal about your life's purpose. Periodically, re-evaluate aspects of your life and make changes that reflect your new awareness.

4 - **Continuing to learn.** Practice new skills at home or work. For example: learn to dance, cook, or fix basic household problems. Take a class on site or online. Dig into that hobby you've been thinking about. Study a new language.

5 - **Savoring life's small pleasures.** Paying attention to even the briefest joyful moments offers opportunities for renewal. Pause to truly notice life's small pleasures: the first flowers of spring, the sun shining through clouds, a moment to offer kindness to a friend.

6 - **Recalling a pleasant or meaningful situation from your past**, an experience that made you smile, experience higher purpose, feel joyful or more fully alive. Savor those thoughts and feelings you experienced and reignite your joy (Fredrickson, 2009).

7 – **Embracing flexibility or discovering new solutions.** If the way you approach a problem isn't working, try a new strategy. Identify the problem, brainstorm ideas to solve it, examine each possibility, and select a solution to try. Anticipating problems and flexibility in resolving them can feel good and build greater meaning.

This week I will notice opportunities to experience greater joy and meaning in my life and my relationships.

CHAPTER 21

Tribute to My Teacher:
A Gratitude Letter

Occasionally, a person comes into our lives who makes a powerful, positive difference. Have you ever had a relationship with a teacher, friend, family member, colleague, or someone else who believed in you and helped you learn to believe in yourself?

Here is a letter expressing my thankfulness that I wrote to my high school music teacher and long-time friend:

My Dear Teacher,

I want to share my heartfelt gratitude, the apex of our story that began many years ago when you were my teacher. Our first meeting was in September all those years ago, in Room 329, Beginning Chorus. I was a sophomore in high school, and you were my new teacher. Although I knew next to nothing about singing in a choir, I was an eager student. The first song we learned was *Wade in the Water,* a spiritual I love to this day. My joy of listening to and singing spirituals and all kinds of music clearly began with you.

In class, you had clear expectations. You were funny and kind in a special way. As I came to know you, you were especially kind to me, and I could make you laugh. I knew from the beginning that you were someone I liked.

Soon, it was spring and time for senior choir auditions. I anxiously sang for you. You accepted me as an alto, later to sing in the tenor section.

Some years later you told me you almost didn't include me in the senior choir, but you saw how much I wanted it. Let me remind you that you also said accepting me was one of the best decisions you ever made! Your candid comment remains a guiding light in my memories, one of the most significant thoughts anyone has ever shared with me. It nurtured my strengths and self-efficacy, made me feel significant and cared about, and let me know you liked me for who I was. I felt you truly saw me and who I could become.

As a junior and senior, I would walk all over the winding hallways of that old three-story school building to find you, just to talk for a few minutes. On days you were absent, it didn't feel so great to be at school. Sometimes, I would go to the attendance office, saying I didn't feel well, because with your absence I didn't see much reason to be there.

My life would have been very different if you hadn't been so kind, hadn't seen me the way you did. Remember when I told you that I didn't want to go to college? Thank you for insisting that I "must go to college" and making me promise that I would. Four degrees and umteen certifications later, I know you were right. Do you remember that you were one of the people to whom I dedicated my doctoral research project? I studied resilience and the factors that strengthen people to bounce back from life's adversities, citing research about how supportive relationships with adults can buffer children and teens from life's challenges (Rutter, 1993; Werner, 1994). Sounds a lot like my relationship with you during high school. You saw my strengths, held my dreams, generously shared your hope and wisdom, and lent me courage and perspective.

As a young adult, I became a teacher because you were a teacher. I wanted to be like you as I saw you but later realized that wasn't possible. I needed to discover my own gifts and find my own path.

Thank you for letting me hang around you during my high school years—especially as a senior—when you certainly could have been doing other things. Thank you for offering to go out with me on prom night if I didn't get a date! Thank you for signing a full page in my yearbook and writing just what I needed to read. You might recall I sat on the floor behind your desk during your ninth period class, trying not to look like I was watching every word you wrote.

Thank you for listening to my youthful emotions and angst, for seeing strengths that I couldn't see in myself, and for accepting me for who I was. Thank you for being that supportive, caring adult in my life who believed in me in a way that I could feel, who helped me feel loved and hopeful, encouraging me toward my potential.

Inspirations

Can you recall someone who has positively impacted your life? Do you have someone you want to thank? The word *gratitude* stems from the Latin *gratia*, meaning grace or gratefulness. Practicing gratitude is recognized among the world's spiritual and ethical traditions. According to contemporary positive psychology research, gratitude is highly linked with happiness, well-being, and positive emotions (Emmons & McCullough, 2003).

One practice involves writing a gratitude letter to someone who has been especially kind or did something good for you in your life, and then, if possible, personally sharing the letter (Seligman, 2011; Seligman et al., 2005). This person could be anyone, perhaps a family member, friend, teacher, mentor, or colleague.

Consider writing a gratitude letter to that person and, if possible, sharing a gratitude visit. Write your note directly to that person and be specific about what impact they have had on your life. If you are unable to conduct an in-person gratitude visit, perhaps you can email it, or you might choose to share what you wrote with someone else.

This week I will recall someone who has positively impacted my life and find a way to express my gratitude.

CHAPTER 22

Awakening Your Creativity
in Everyday Life

About a year into the lonely days of the COVID pandemic, I decided to pick up my dusty old guitar after years of sporadic, infrequent use. With all the social restrictions, I longed to make music and sing with others. I thought playing my guitar, even with limited skills, would give me a reason to sing and would bring greater joy, meaning, and fulfillment into my days (Berns-Zare, 2022).

Although my guitar abilities had never progressed much beyond a beginner's level, I was game to try, curious and excited about the possibilities. I decided to activate my courage and take a few guitar lessons remotely. Then a few months later, my husband gifted me a new folk guitar for my birthday. Even shopping for the instrument was a novel experiment. Let's just say I was probably the oldest person shopping in the guitar stores I visited. With a friend's help, I chose a Martin guitar with a warm, vibrant tone and potential for beautiful sound well beyond my ability level.

I found that making music with my voice and emerging guitar skills awakened my creativity, perhaps thanks more to my love of music and perseverance than talent. Thus, during the last few years, I've had some good times bolstering my skills, amusing myself, occasionally making music with friends, and experiencing a sense of accomplishment in this season of my life.

I believe that my simple musical efforts enlivened my overall creativity. During the pandemic period, I also tried my hand at baking bread. While the outcome was definitely not as tasty as I'd hoped for, the process itself was filled with sticky hands, joyful moments, and surprisingly meaningful creativity. Spurred by my emerging creative flow, I decided to venture into nonfiction writing. After several years of creative effort and revising, editing, revising and more revising, this book has emerged.

In a mixture of joy, frustration, and anticipation, I believe that while I may not master any of these creative endeavors, I can continue to go with the flow, tapping into my internal resources, and nurturing my inspiration, interests, imagination and creative wellspring. Sometimes, I become so immersed in the reverie of the creative process that I lose track of time. This deep absorption and enjoyment of an everyday experience has been termed *flow* and can contribute to our wellbeing and fulfillment (Csikszentmihaly, 1990; Kaufman, 2020).

Your creativity can grow as you tap it, play with it, and practice it. The brain is truly remarkable in its abilities to adapt, combine, and transform accumulated resources in fresh, new ways, forming new connections in a process called *neuroplasticity* (Beaty, 2020; Kennedy & Gonzalez, 2023). This ability to develop fresh connections with new experiences and ideas is pivotal to creativity of all kinds.

The terms *everyday creativity* or *small-c creativity* are used to describe openness to new experiences and originality in daily life (Richards, 2007; Simonton, 2001). Children are naturally creative in this way. As an adult, you can also cultivate your inventiveness, ideas, and expressiveness, particularly every day, small-c creativity.

Regardless of external events, you can pay attention to and experiment with daily occurrences, quiet inklings, and the savoring of experiences in the moment. Creative awakening need not result in any product but may simply involve the intention and process of opening to new or unexpected experiences. Creative processes invite you to reduce self-judgement and rigidity, embracing possibilities with what the Buddhists call *beginners mind.*

A contributor to the creative process is a *growth mindset,* a concept discussed in Chapter 8 of this book. Embracing a growth mindset involves a belief that you can learn from your missteps and with hard work and good strategies you can develop your abilities (Dweck, 2006, 2016). A growth mindset can support creative energies, efforts, and motivations, springboarding achievements in life.

You might be surprised to learn that creativity is common. Everyone has some creative capacity. In fact, creativity is one of the 24 character strengths common to humankind across all cultures (Niemiec, 2014). The concepts shared in this chapter are *not* about creative genius, rather they are about welcoming creativity in the context of your everyday life. Each day is an opportunity to invite yourself to think about things in new ways, generating new ideas and possibilities, and then notice what happens.

Inspirations

What if you experimented with greater openness, flexibility, and creative expression in your everyday experience? There are many ways to integrate creative processes into day-to-day life, whether for moments or hours.

Here are 21 ways to awaken creativity in your everyday life. This week, play with one or two creative ideas that interest you.

1. Travel to a new location, whether locally or beyond, or travel to a familiar location using a different route or mode of transportation.
2. Brainstorm novel (different) ways to do a task, even an everyday chore.
3. Grow a few plants in your window or start a small garden.
4. Use a common object, such as a mug or plastic container in a novel, new way. For example, decorate a coffee mug with stickers or paint; use a cup as a planter or pen/pencil holder; or brainstorm alternative uses for a plastic or cardboard container.
5. Try a new hobby or leisure activity.
6. Make up a poem, rhyme, or riddle just for fun.

7. At work or at home, try doing an everyday task with your non-dominant hand.

8. Do a painting project, wood project or fix something that's broken.

9. After you listen to a podcast or read a book or article, record some of your reactions in your notebook or on your electronic device.

10. Rearrange some of the furniture or items in your living space.

11. Pick up that knitting, sewing, or needlework project you've been thinking about.

12. Ponder a creative solution to an everyday problem and, if feasible, give it a try.

13. Play with a child or talk with a teenager in your life.

14. Sing in the car or the shower.

15. Have fun working on your dance moves or simply engage in some creative movement.

16. Attend a concert, show, or play on site or virtually.

17. Doodle on paper with pencil, pen, or markers.

18. Learn a musical instrument or try drumming on a book or a counter.

19. Write a letter or email to a friend, create a poem, or begin jotting notes for a book you've always wanted to write.

20. Share some reminiscences or some of your life experiences with a younger person who might be interested.

21. Play a game that encourages you to think creatively, like Scrabble, Dominoes, Chess, or Charades.

This week I will tap into my creativity and notice how it feels.

CHAPTER 23

Listening with a Hearing Heart

I took my 5-year-old granddaughter to see a movie in which one of the female heroines, trying to figure out what to do in a difficult situation, asked the question, "What is the next right thing?" (Anderson-Lopez & Lopez, 2019).

This weighty question stuck with me. And then a few weeks later at a study session, another question got my attention: "How do I know I'm doing the right thing?" In my second half of life wanderings, these inquiries have awakened me as I reflect on and respond to my own life's questions. There is so much noise in my own head and in the world around me, and yet sometimes when I listen carefully, I experience an interior sense of much more (Berns-Zare, 2020b).

How do we ask, listen to, and respond to life's important questions? Spiritual director Barbara Breitman (2006) writes that we don't only hear with our ears but also with our hearts. She calls it the "hearing heart." Perhaps in some moments, we have opportunities to engage in deeper, fuller forms of listening. And what do we hear? Perhaps, as we listen more deeply, we may notice moments of clarity or insights that shine greater light on how we can live.

So, how do we explore whether we're doing the right thing in any given situation? And how do we figure out what the next right thing might be? Each of us comes to our connection with what we value and life's universal truths on our own terms. Each of us is responsible for deciding how these truths may manifest in our life's choices. Perhaps there are many *right* paths, each offering different teachings, learnings, and outcomes.

I suspect that love is the universal and very human underlying current in our day-to-day lives and that when love filters our choices and decisions, we're more prepared to pause, ask, listen to, and respond to life's questions.

Love is not just a modern cliché. As you read in Chapter 20, the good feelings emanating from connection are hardwired into our human biology, potentially igniting positive emotions when we relate to others. The human body's cells physiologically respond to love, releasing chemicals such as the hormone oxytocin, which plays a major role in attachment and social bonding (Fredrickson, 2013). The experience of love helps to shield us from illness and leads us toward health and flourishing, amplifying the practical, physical, and spiritual aspects of who we are—mind, body, and spirit. Love can bind us with each other, affecting who we are and who we can become. Love can enliven us to truly experience ourselves and others with kindness, care, and compassion. Isn't it interesting how love can benefit our health and well-being, the actual biology of our bodies?

Think about it. Babies come into the world hungry for love and connection. They instinctively seek relationships through eye contact and even synchronize their movements with caregivers, for example, smiling when we smile. Children and adults seek love in intimate partnerships, friendships, and communities. And researchers have discovered *mirror neurons* in the human brain (Ramchandran, 2011). These mirror neurons indicate that we are biologically designed so that our brains synchronize as we connect with each other to the extent that during positive communications people may experience a single shared emotion that syncs or connects between their brains.

So, how can we figure out "What's the next right thing" and "How do I know I'm doing the right thing?" And let's add one more question we might ask ourselves in any given situation: "What would love do?"

Inspirations

This week consider the balance between listening, reflection, and action, as you gently notice your hearing heart. I invite you to experiment with one or both of these inspirational practices.

Practice 1 – Listening to your own inner stirrings with a hearing heart.

Create a moment in your day to pause. Notice that you are breathing. Gently invite your attention to rest there for a moment. Now, consider an issue in your life and invite yourself to ponder one or more of these questions:

- What's on my mind or my heart right now?
- Is this something I want to contemplate, reflect on, or take an action about?
- What is the next right thing?
- How do I know I am doing the right thing?
- What would love do?

You might experiment with listening deeply to your contemplations not only with your ears but also with your inner essence, with your heart. Can you offer yourself gentle gifts of self-compassion and love as you pause to notice what arises for you? Can you listen to whispers of the quiet voice within you?

Let love light your way as you reflect on the wisdom of your experiences, your learnings, your values, and your own inner compass.

Invite yourself to gently notice whatever comes to awareness. Perhaps you might notice not only what is visible but also the roots below the surface?

What are you aware of that perhaps you hadn't noticed before?

Practice 2 – Reflecting on phrases of lovingkindness.

This compassionate meditation practice, which has evolved from Buddhist origins, can help you open your heart, feel more interconnected, and create a habit of goodwill toward others (Fredrickson, 2013; Salzburg, 2010).

In a quiet moment, settle into an awareness of the flow of your breathing or other anchor such as your feet touching the floor or a sound in your environment.

You might reflect on a few simple lovingkindness phrases, directing them first toward yourself. Examples of compassionate phrases include: "May I be safe;" "May I be well;" "May I be happy;" "May I be at peace."

When you're ready, you might reflect on lovingkindness phrases directed toward a particular person you know well and then toward one or more acquaintances—or toward the world in general. May you be safe; may you be well; may you be happy; may you be at peace.

As you complete your loving-kindness practice, what do you notice?

**_This week I will take a few moments each day
to pause, listen with my hearing heart, and ponder
life's questions._**

CHAPTER 24

Our Beliefs and Self-Empowerment
to Create Change

Some years ago, I led a multi-community coalition for prevention of substance abuse in at-risk youth and communities. My role involved many challenging responsibilities, and at times I felt that I was not up to meeting them. An older, wiser colleague inspired me to reflect on what I believed about my capabilities and potential and what impact my beliefs had on my thoughts and behaviors. Over time, adopting the practice of naming my beliefs and confronting those assumptions that no longer served me well positively shifted how I saw challenges, adversities, and my capacity to respond.

How powerful is belief? Our beliefs can be personal assumptions so natural to us that sometimes we are not even aware of their existence within us. According to Esther Sternberg, a leading neuroscience expert, our beliefs, assumptions, and deep convictions have many aspects, but their basis is *learning* (2001). And our beliefs not only affect our thinking, but they can also influence our perceptions, the decisions we make, and the actions we choose, such as how we take care of ourselves, how we interact with others, and how we respond to events within our environment. We carry these assumptions and associations with us whether we are aware of them or not. For example, when you try something new, what do you believe could happen? Do you typically experience feelings of excitement, hope, worry, confusion, pressure, or something else?

Research in neuroscience, the scientific study of the brain and nervous system, shows that the human brain changes, grows, and forms new connections as we learn throughout our lives. Young or old, as we learn, our brains continue to change, making new connections among experiences, emotions, and behaviors. When we learn something new, the pathways in our brains form new associations in a process called *neuroplasticity*. Thus, our beliefs, understandings, thoughts, behaviors, and new learnings actually change us. As we shift our beliefs, we enable new associations between where we are now and where we want to be.

In many ways, our beliefs frame who we are and who we become. We are participants in creating our own realities. At any stage of life, our thoughts, beliefs, and attitudes influence how we respond to our experiences.

While we may not have much control over external events, we do have choices about paying attention to our beliefs and how we relate to what happens to us and in our world.

- We can have an impact on the story we tell ourselves about whatever has happened, and we can edit that story.
- We can choose how we respond within ourselves and with others. For example, do we respond with anger, impatience, and divisiveness or with kindness, patience, and deep listening?
- We can choose to *not* believe an inner critic that tells us we are flawed. We can disagree with that critic, set it aside, and use our experiences as opportunities to reflect and edit our beliefs, search for meaning, and develop a greater acceptance of ourselves and others.
- When we are ready, we can choose to take actions to transform our beliefs into realities.

Inspirations

Here are some ideas you may want to experiment with:

1 - Pay attention to your beliefs and recognize how they affect your experience. Notice the messages and stories you tell yourself. You have

choices about your self-talk, so why not choose inspiring messages that bolster positive emotions, strengths, and well-being? Invite yourself to shift your beliefs when you feel it would benefit you.

2 - Reframe how you think about one or more situations. There is more than one way to look at most of them. If you see yourself locked in a negative belief or perspective, can you open your mind to broadened possibilities and other options? Reframing invites you to view a situation differently. A new approach can inspire growth, alternative actions, and improve your well-being.

3 - Consider the connection between your beliefs about adversity and your emotional and behavioral responses. Some programs in positive psychology are based on the ABC model (Ellis, 1997; Seligman, 2011), which emphasizes that our beliefs about *Adversity* cause the feelings we experience. When something happens, we create an explanation about what happened and why, and these *Beliefs* influence our reactions or *Consequences*.

For example, let's say you set a goal to walk five days weekly for 30 minutes. For two weeks you meet your goal. During the third week you walk three times, and the fourth week you walk only twice. If your belief is that you never finish anything you start and this is an example of another personal failure, you might give up trying to achieve your goal. However, if you believe this is a minor setback and you know that setbacks are part of creating behavior change you may choose to renew your efforts and continue to work toward your goal.

4 - Learn to notice the positives. Create time to pause each day. Make a mental or written note of the positives and successes of the day, large and small.

This week I will pay attention to my beliefs and empower myself to consider where I am currently and how I hope to show up in my life.

CHAPTER 25

What Story Are You Writing with Your Unique and Precious Life?

As we navigate midlife and beyond, we are stakeholders not only in the present but also in the future. Our choices infuse our days and affect those around us, carrying implications for today, tomorrow, and future generations.

You may recall psychologist Abraham Maslow's 5-stage model, a pyramid describing the hierarchy of needs (1943;1987). The model suggests that all of us have a natural desire toward self-actualization, i.e. fulfilling our highest potential in life. Although there is no script, Maslow proposed that to approach self-actualization, we need to satisfy needs ranging from basic to more complex: physiological (food, water, rest, air), safety, love and belonging, and esteem (from others and for ourselves). As we grow and learn, while still maintaining relationships and respecting others, we can move toward our unique and precious potential, the best version of ourselves: self-actualization. This stage is *not* about perfection; rather, it involves engaging our strengths, capacities, potential, and the desire to take steps toward growing into our best selves. As we hit our stride at midlife and beyond, many of us aspire toward self-actualization, seeking greater awareness of life's meanings, interconnections, and values. We seek to make contributions to the world, doing the best we are capable of in this season of our lives.

Our lives are works in progress. Waking up each day, we create our own stories. Realizing that any story, no matter who creates it, contains the viewpoint of the writer, offers us precious possibilities to explore our aliveness. We have opportunities to awaken in new ways, reinventing aspects of ourselves as we reflect on and reimagine our next chapters and our relationships within the world in which we live.

Your life unfolds each day, inviting you to wake up to your internal voice, to open toward your possibilities, to new chronicles waiting to be created and shared. As you consider your own story, you can reflect on what you're doing, what you've learned, and who you are becoming each day. What are your strengths, your longings, your actions, and contributions? Where have you been, where are you currently, and what are your next steps? Where do you feel inspired or called, and how will you answer the call?

Inspirations

Take some time to explore your own story, the narrative of your unique and precious life. Pay attention to your heart, your intuition, your life experiences, your wisdom, and your observations from the world around you.

Here are some questions you might consider:

- How am I developing toward my unique and precious potential?
- How can I engage my wisdom, creativity, and life experiences as I write the next chapter of my life?
- How do I navigate my strengths and my vulnerability in this lifetime?
- How can I live with greater authenticity, compassion, and meaning?
- Am I contributing to life's problems or solutions?
- Am I creating a positive footprint in the world—no matter how small or large?
- How can I contribute toward caring for and repairing the brokenness in our world?

- What is my legacy thus far? What would I like my legacy to become?
- How might my story bring me more deeply toward myself as I explore my unique potential in this season of my life.

This week I will consider my own story and think about how I want to write my next chapter.

CHAPTER 26

Discovering Greater Resilience, Connection, and Common Ground

Although we live our lives as if we were separate entities, scientific findings and teachings of many spiritual traditions declare that we are all interconnected. Science continues to discover that humanity is part of the interconnected wholeness of the universe (Swimme & Berry, 1992). In visible and invisible ways, we are *all* part of the great whole. We humans all share the same common ground, the earth, which is a small fraction of a vast and ever-expanding universe. We are forever connected with each other and the continually unfolding infinite aspects of life.

Each of us has much to share with humanity. Our voices matter. Our choices matter. And although we are unique individuals, our presence along with our decisions, actions, and inactions are an integral part of the collective oneness of our communities and our world.

At times, such complex ideas can feel overwhelming. In our vulnerability and humanity, we naturally compartmentalize, viewing things from our own individual perspectives and vantage points. Typically, we map out our territory, fencing ourselves in and others out so that we feel safe and protected with some sense of control over the many uncertainties that confront us.

There are no simple answers to the labyrinth of issues that contribute to the wholeness and brokenness in our world, and I certainly don't claim to have them. One of my beliefs is that embracing our inherent interconnectedness is not about seeking perfection but an invitation to embrace our struggles, feelings of disconnection, and brokenness as part of living. Life invites us to ask ourselves how we can embrace our challenges as opportunities to grow and seek common ground (Palmer, 2024).

When we divide ourselves against the *other*, we may neglect the many commonalities that naturally bind us together. When we divide ourselves against the other, we may create conflict that denies the wholeness of our interdependence, the universal life force that gives us breath, and our indomitable spirits. Philosopher and social activist Vimala Thakar notes that with awareness of our wholeness, we can develop toward greater understanding that each moment and each action is meaningful (1984).

Yes, the words we choose make a difference. Our actions and inactions matter. Some conversations and actions can be meaningful and life-changing in ways that can create connection or damage connection. How can we navigate difficult conversations with kindness and resilience? How do we get back up when we fall down, when tensions are high, or when we misstep or say or do the wrong thing, whether inadvertently or purposefully?

It's a slippery slope to be careless about what we say and how we say it, to be careless about what we do and what we don't do. Impulsive actions and reactions and our shifting emotions can leave us feeling isolated, divided, lost, and less connected to others (Brown, 2021). Sometimes, rash, mindless words and actions slip out quickly and reflexively before we can pause and think about their impact and consequences. We may in the moment choose the most convenient phrase or a harsh word, but if we pause briefly to create space between our experience and our response, we might make a different choice (Frankl, 1984; Goleman & Boyatzis, 2017). With a pause and more thought, foresight, or kindness, we can choose to express our ideas, feelings, or actions more mindfully.

How do we get back up when we have made choices that we now see differently? How do we seek common ground when great distances divide us? For some of us, this arena of resilience may involve a sense of ourselves as part of something larger, part of the interconnected wholeness of our world. As humans, we are inherently resilient. We have the capacity to respond to and recover from life's adversities – to adjust, learn, and move forward from our experiences.

Resilience is a commonality among us, ordinary, rather than extraordinary (American Psychological Association, 2014; Egeland et al., 1993). We can view resilience as a toolbox of skills that we can learn, practice, strengthen, and expand. Resilience is not about bouncing back; it's about going forward from where we find ourselves. When things we're doing aren't working, a resilient mindset can inspire us to ask and respond to questions such as *"What can I do differently?"* and *"How can I move forward from this situation?"* Leaning into our resilience and employing the many strategies that strengthen resilience can empower us to shift from the confinements of our challenges to a sense of agency, knowing that we have choices in how we respond (Bandura, 1997).

Humans have faced the challenges of feeling connected and disconnected throughout our history. We have faced difficult challenges of many kinds and responded to them. Indeed, we humans have the capacity to be quite resilient—to grow, change, act, and evolve in ways that contribute toward repairing and healing this world.

Inspirations

Here are three approaches to help you reach more deeply into yourself and engage with others, whether or not they see things the way you do. These approaches may help you discover a path toward greater resilience through connectedness within yourself and with others in this interconnected world:

Approach 1 – *Where are you?* You may experience greater calm, compassion, and effectiveness when you approach your interactions and your life more mindfully (Goleman & Davidson, 2017). You can strengthen your resilience skills by realizing where you are and training yourself to react with greater mindfulness, ease, and calm. Here are four simple steps:

- Step A: Create a pause for a moment in a quiet, safe place.
- Step B: Take a comfortable deep breath and slowly release it.
- Step C: Notice what's happening in your body and mind. See if you can just notice and soften into it. No need to judge anything.
- Step D: Take another comfortably slow, deep breath and feel your body begin to relax.

Approach 2 – *How can you reach across differences that divide?* Adrian Michael Green (2019) offers these tools to help us navigate our differences when we have difficult conversations:

- Listen to people. Strive to meet people where they are rather than jumping into what you think and want to say.
- Give people room to speak, trying not to take the things they say personally. Give the other person and yourself the chance "to be messy," to reflect, and to clarify.
- Strive to build bridges, not barriers.
- Don't hide from discomfort more than you need to. Instead, as you are able, lean into uncomfortable conversations, really listening to what people have to say, noticing and labeling your emotions, and noticing what's happening in your body in an effort to stay in the present moment.
- Before discussions or meetings, create a bit of common ground with the other participant(s). It can help to set norms so that participants can agree on how they might respond if the conversation gets tense or becomes difficult.

Approach 3 – *How can you invite others toward common ground?* These ideas are inspired by the life of Supreme Court Justice Ruth Bader Ginsberg, who encouraged people to stand up for what matters. Importantly, Ginsberg challenged us to think before we speak and encouraged dialogue in a way that respects the humanity of others even those with differing beliefs (Breyer, 2020-2021; Duehren, 2015; Ginsberg, 2016; Tyler, 2020-2021).

- Listen quietly and respectfully.
- Before you speak, think carefully about your words, and choose them wisely.
- Choose your words wisely when you speak or write.
- Be an active voice for calm, reason, and respecting others.
- Stand up for what's important while also building relationships and valuing others whether you agree or disagree.
- Continue to learn and grow throughout your lifetime: take care of your body, your mind, and your spirit.

This week I will practice being present and responding with greater mindfulness, wisdom, and calm.

CHAPTER 27

Reflection, Discernment, and Transformation

One day, I was bemoaning the inevitable passing of time in my life. A wise friend, a decade ahead of me in years and life experience, reminded me that each day offers priceless opportunities, that any day can bring joys, challenges, and possibilities. As a result, I have developed an awareness that while we may not have much control over external events and the challenges that life serves up, we do have influence over our choices, how we respond, and what we might learn from our experiences.

Not long ago, feeling swamped with a full schedule, I thought I'd get a few things done at the same time. With two hardcover books under my arm and an electronic device in hand, I also picked up a glass of tea and a chunk of dark chocolate to carry to my table so I could scan email while I snacked. No surprise, the glass dropped, shattering into what seemed like a thousand pieces across the ceramic floor. Rather than saving 15 seconds, my choice to heedlessly multi-task resulted in 15 unhappy *minutes* spent cleaning up the glass and tea from the floor.

What did I learn from this experience? From the many possible options in this simple situation, I chose to do several things all at once. Hopefully, next time I might make a different choice. Reflecting on our experiences and learning from them can continue throughout our lives. No two people are exactly alike and for each of us our paths are different and greatly influenced by our choices, decisions, and actions.

Each day we face challenges, transitions, and new possibilities. Some of us try to do too much. Sometimes, we feel stuck, lost, or worried. Or we may feel that something is missing in our lives. Or we may desire to live with greater authenticity, spontaneity, or purpose.

Rather than staying stuck or looking for magic answers somewhere *out there*, how can you discern a transformative path toward your next steps? How can you learn to live from the inside out, honoring your own truths in the light of external events and life's big picture?

Drawing on ideas from positive psychology, mindfulness, and neuroscience along with mind, body, and spiritual integrative practices, this chapter offers a personal discernment process to help you re-energize and gain clarity as you discover your next steps on life's journey.

The **PARDA 5-Step Awakening and Action Process** encompasses five integral steps (Berns-Zare, 2020c; 2023a; 2025).

1. **<u>Pause</u>** and mindfully focus on the quiet flow of your breathing or another calming home base for your attention.

2. **<u>Actively Listen</u>** to your intuition and inner voice. In the pause you've created, tune into the still small voice and inner compass that guides you.

3. **<u>Reflect</u>** on your experience. With self-compassion, listen to messages from your thoughts, feelings, and bodily sensations.

4. **<u>Discern</u>** as you sift through your awareness, intuitive wisdom, realities, possibilities, and choices.

5. **<u>Act</u>** mindfully and with intention, choosing your next steps for reflection or action.

> **Pause. Listen. Reflect. Discern.**
> **Act mindfully to choose your next steps.**

Inspirations

Now you can invite yourself to pause, pay attention, reflect, and choose your next steps. These five steps can help you guide your personal exploration.

1. Pause: Create an intermission in your day. Offer yourself a few moments of quiet contemplation to help you tune into your inner voice.

Make sure you're in a safe space. Then, invite yourself to get into a comfortable position and focus on a calming anchor, or home base, for the wandering mind, such as your breath, your hands, an image around you, or a sound in the environment. Many people choose the breath as it's portable and always with you. You may want to gently put a hand on your heart space or abdomen.

Gently become aware that you are breathing (or pay attention to whatever anchor you have chosen). If breath is your anchor, simply notice your breath as it flows in and out of your body, breathing mindfully as you meet the moment. If it feels safe to you, you might close your eyes softly or leave them open resting them on the floor in front of you. Pause here, noticing the flow of your breathing (or other anchor) for a brief time if that feels right to you.

2. Actively Listen: In the pause you've created, invite yourself to listen deeply within you. Pay attention to messages from your mind, body, and spirit. What are you noticing on your mind and in your heart, or as a "gut feeling"? Gently observe where your attention gravitates and let yourself be present where you are called in this moment. Open to your inner knowing, your intuition, and your values. What are you sensing with your inner compass or guide?

3. Reflect: What are you noticing about how you feel? Are you excited, content, sad, worried, hurt, resentful, angry, hopeful, happy, or other emotions? Try to name the feeling or feelings for yourself. What are you noticing in your body? What is your experience?

What might your inner voice of guidance and wisdom be letting you know? What do you know deep inside yourself that perhaps you don't often let yourself pay attention to? What are you sensing with your inner compass or guide?

Perhaps an image, a hunch, a fleeting feeling, or a knowing is waiting there for you to become aware of.

4. Discern: Listen, hear, see, and/or feel what is coming into your awareness. Consider self-inquiries such as:

- Where do I feel inspiration? For example: energy, joy, understanding, happiness, openness, gratitude, zest?
- Where do I feel desolation? Such as: frustration, confusion, anger, restlessness, sadness, meaninglessness?
- What seems most significant for me to pay attention to right now?
- Where do I feel called?
- What do I want to reject or move away from?
- What can I release or let go of?
- What beckons to me to move toward it?
- What am I aware of now that I hadn't noticed or let myself see before?

Act mindfully with intention: What has shifted for you during this process? What are you learning about yourself or the situation? What, if any, direction do you want to go toward? What do you want to continue to reflect on and where might you want to take action? What is your next right step?

*This week I will contemplate a positive shift in my life as
I pause, listen, reflect, discern, and mindfully choose
my next steps.*

CHAPTER 28

Which Path Will You Choose?

As I write this chapter, I am sitting in my yard, noticing the changes that fall brings. Although most trees have shed their leaves, the white-trunked river birch in the corner of our garden continues to carry most of its bright golden leaves. An avid gardener, I am aware that it is time to put the garden to bed in preparation for winter. With quiet, colder temperatures, and a sleepy winter's rest, the garden can flourish when spring bursts forth.

For many of us, fall is a time of transition, a gateway of opportunity to review the adventures of summer and look ahead toward new beginnings. Some of us jump quickly into the next venture. We may have a vision for what's next, and we're ready to get started. Others may feel sadness, grieving the loss of summer's warm meandering days. While some of us may not welcome the cooler season, we learn to live with its changes, letting the flow of daily life carry us toward next steps.

I am reminded of the words of Holocaust survivor Viktor Frankl. In his remarkable book, *Man's Search for Meaning*, Frankl shared how he survived the brutality of Holocaust concentration camps by finding meaning in even the most difficult circumstances (1959, 1985). Frankl wrote about freedom, the space that exists between a stimulus (an event) and our response to it. He emphasized our capacity, in any circumstance, to choose how we will answer. Frankl taught that our ability to grow toward freedom can be discovered in how we respond to the circumstances that life throws at us.

These ideas continue to hold significance for us today. Frankl did *not* believe there were simple answers to life's difficult questions. Rather, he wrote that within any circumstance, even when we are suffering with life's most grueling challenges, we have the freedom to make choices about how we will respond. This realization is fundamental to how we can approach and transcend difficulties and find our way toward greater meaning in our lives.

Thus, between what happens and how you answer it, you have more freedom than you may realize. Freedom to pause. Freedom to reflect. Freedom to choose your attitude and how you respond. What stories do you tell yourself about happenings in your life, e.g. "this is a good thing" or "this is a bad thing;" "I like this" or "this stinks." You can derive greater meaning and personal growth by embracing your freedom of choice, reflecting on your attitude about life's events and how you choose to respond to them.

Inspirations

Consider a situation that you are facing currently. This practice offers a framework you can draw on as you approach your options and choices in a wide range of situations.

An 8-Step Approach for Choosing Your Path:

Step 1. Pause to intentionally create space between the situation and your response. Take a few conscious breaths and with each breath, you may notice the flow of the air as you inhale and then exhale. Or, as discussed in Chapter 27, you may prefer to choose an alternate anchor for your attention, such as your hands, your feet touching the ground, or an image. As you observe your breaths, you might focus on one of these simple phrases. *Breathe in love, breathe out fear. Breathe in freedom, breathe out limitation. I am breathing in, I am breathing out.*

Step 2. Clearly identify the situation. Be specific. It may help to write information about the situation in your journal, notebook, or notes on your electronic device.

Step 3. Consider your goals for resolving the situation. Again, you may want to write down your goal(s).

Step 4. Brainstorm some ideas and possibilities for solutions. Write these ideas down as well.

Step 5. Assess the ideas. Seek more information, support, or resources as needed.

Step 6. Choose the solution/response that you think best fits the situation.

Step 7. Take any actions you decide on.

Step 8. Evaluate the outcomes.

This week I will intentionally reflect on a situation I am facing and consider which path I may choose.

CHAPTER 29

Rituals and Meaningful
Everyday Practices

Our contemporary, multifaceted lives are peppered with traditions, rites of passage, ceremonies, celebrations. Some rituals are imbued with compelling meaning, while others may feel like obligations forced by pressures of family, work, organizations, or other sources.

Many rituals filter across the seasons of our lives and can help us connect within ourselves, unite with each other, and relate to the natural world and beyond (Berns-Zare, 2024). Across time and place, group rituals are unifying behaviors whether in cultural, religious, and spiritual traditions or academics, sports, workplaces, the military, or other organizations. And as individuals, many of us engage in practices that we may imbue with connotations and significance that bring meaning, purpose and mattering into our lives.

Yet, rituals differ from routines. Many habits and routines are merely activities we repeat regularly, while rituals can have meanings or purpose that in some way extend beyond the tasks themselves (Hobson, et al., 2024; Norton, 2024; Smith & Steward, 2011). Sometimes we create our own rituals and meaningful practices. I have a friend whose preparation of her afternoon coffee break and snack is a meaningful ritual activity. Several days a week, she prepares her beverage carefully and lovingly, making certain each step is performed exactly as she prefers. For my friend, this activity offers a satisfying and meaningful way to create a pause in her day as she sits down to savor her treat and mindfully enjoy moments of quiet contemplation.

When we choose to include an attitude of mindfulness, savoring, or gratitude, even simple rituals can offer enlivening rhythms that percolate through our day-to-day existence. Participating in existing rituals and creating or re-creating our own can help us bring more meaning and wellbeing into our lives.

Engaging in rituals in ways that feel personally meaningful can contribute to our sense of *mattering*. That is, feeling that we are visible and significant in some way, such as experiencing connection to others interpersonally or as part of a larger whole (Flett, 2022; Kellerman & Seligman, 2023), e.g., volunteering at an annual community event, participating in a group ritual with a religious organization, or engaging in a social action or political process. Mattering and feeling appreciated by others can be important across the span of our lives and may be noteworthy to consider during important transitions, such as a job change, major life event, or retirement.

With creativity and intention, you can choose to transform a mundane, everyday activity or routine into a ritual imbued with a sense of meaning. In his book, *The Power of Ritual*, Casper Ter Kuile, describes engaging with rituals to create meaning at four levels of connection: connecting with oneself, connecting with other people, connecting with the natural world, and connecting with something that feels transcendent or somehow larger than yourself or ordinary activity (2020).

Inspirations

While some rituals feel calming, others may energize, inspire, or help you feel part of something larger than yourself. For example, some people have a morning routine with an intention of creating motivation and inspiration. When you wake up, do you jump quickly out of bed, or do you pause with gratitude for a new day, maybe offering a brief meditation, prayer, or pondering something you are grateful for? In the evening, do you quickly read a story to the child in your life before bed so you can get to the next task, or do you share a meaningful bedtime ritual, such as reading the story, discussing it, and talking about its meaning?

You can empower yourself to rebuild a habit or task into a purposeful, meaningful or sacred ritual. The key is how you feel about this practice and what you are thinking about when you engage with it. Which rituals in your life do you find most meaningful? How could you explore an existing ritual, design a new meaningful everyday ritual, or adapt an older one that you have ignored or let go of?

Here are some rituals you might want to consider:

Personal rituals:

- Meaningful or sacred reading as a pathway to greater awareness.
- Pausing for a moment of mindfulness or reflection about how you want to be present before an important meeting or event.
- Taking a beloved youth out for lunch each year before the first day of school to discuss aspirational goals for the year.
- Noticing a significant life passage with a simple personal ceremony, such as lighting a candle, planting some seeds, or a moment of silence.
- Taking time out from working or daily tasks in an intentional way to rest and rejuvenate.

Rituals with others:

- Planting a community garden with other people each spring.
- Connecting with others in intentional companionship, whether taking a walk, a weekly phone conversation, or sharing a monthly dinner together.
- Preparing meals with family or friends at certain holidays.
- A community healing ceremony after a loss.
- Celebrating birthdays by lighting candles and singing.
- Participating in graduations, sun dances, spiritual ceremonies or other community celebrations.

Rituals engaging with the natural world:

- Celebrating the new moon or full moon each month.
- Harvesting fruits and vegetables with gratitude for the bounty.
- Regularly noticing nature by spending time in a garden, wooded area or near water.
- Sitting silently with reverence to watch the sunrise or sunset.

Transcendent Rituals:

- Participating in spiritual ceremonies and practices, such as contemplating blessings, gratitude, or observing significant holidays or traditions, whether on your own or as part of a community.
- Coming of age ceremonies to celebrate rites of passage, such as confirmations, b'nei mitzvahs,[1] and communions.
- Attending funerals or other memorial observances.

How might engaging in ritual enrich your life? What everyday activity might you want to transform into a simple ritual to bring greater meaning into your life?

***This week I will think about the role of meaningful rituals and everyday practices in my life.
Is there something I want to add or change to create greater meaning?***

---

1 A bnei mitzvah is a Jewish symbolic ritual marking the passage from childhood to adulthood, greater learning, and service.

CHAPTER 30

Reimagining Possibilities
for Aging Well

To be alive is to be growing older. What are your assumptions about possibilities for living a fulfilling life into your next decades? Do you view aging through a positive lens with evolving potential for change, new learning, and growth opportunities, or do you view it primarily through a negative frame as a time of inevitable, uncontrollable decline?

How might you challenge your assumptions about longevity that don't serve you well, as you redefine aging and reimagine your own possibilities for growing older with greater wellbeing? What factors may help you live more resiliently into mid-life and later life?

In a remarkable study on self-perceptions of longevity and aging, Yale University researcher Becca Levy, a leading authority on how beliefs about getting older influence aging, found that adults who held more positive views on elderhood lived 7.5 years longer than people with more negative views (Levy et al., 2002). In other words, our views on getting older can influence longevity and wellbeing.

This information invites us to pay attention to our beliefs about how we think about aging and our passage through the years. Sometimes, we may not be aware of some of the stereotypes about aging that influence us. Deciphering our expectations and beliefs about what it means to grow older can help us approach our health and well-being with greater self-empowerment and can influence how we age. More positive expectations and perceptions can yield more positive outcomes in ways that can extend our health and longevity (Langer, 2009; Levy et al., 2002).

Aging well involves two important aspects. One is lifespan, how long you live. The other component has been termed *health span*, relating to your quality of life and living as well as you can (Attia, 2023). A powerful approach is to pay mindful attention to your body, noticing how you feel and exploring varied possibilities for your health and wellbeing. By being highly involved in your own self-care and navigating strategies for well-being, you can empower yourself as you consider your current and future pathways. Harvard researcher Ellen Langer (2017) recommends actions such as becoming attuned to the variability in your body and vigorously advocating for yourself. For example, you can notice how you feel, explore what the reasons might be, and ask questions not only of your healthcare and wellness partners but also of yourself.

Inspirations

This week, thoughtfully consider your current views on getting older with wellbeing in each season of your life. What are your assumptions about longevity and aging? How might you challenge expectations that may be untrue or that don't suit you? Remember that aging well involves a focus on social, emotional, spiritual, and physical health (Vaillant, 2002). Does your current awareness and lifestyle nurture all four of these areas? Would one of them benefit from greater focus?

Answers about ways to bolster your wellbeing are *not* one-size-fits-all. Perhaps a key question is "How can I live better in this season of my life and in the seasons to come?" As you choose to fortify your wellbeing toolbox, you may notice that health and illness are often not either-or propositions. Rather, health, wellbeing, and fulfillment exist on a complex and varied continuum, offering possibilities for revised understanding, opportunities, and choice-points along the way. Let a mindful approach to your wellbeing, decisions, and choices guide you toward living the best life you can. Here are a few ideas:

- Continue to learn about yourself and about strategies to help you live *your* best life.
- Pay attention to what your heart and inner compass are letting you know.
- Seek out accurate and relevant information about healthy lifestyle options and practices, preventing illness, and intervening early before minor issues become more serious.
- Ask lots of questions (there are no dumb questions).
- Consider the role of mindfulness as a practice to inspire and fortify your well-being and positive aging.
- Consult with experts and resources as needed.
- Identify advocates and supports with whom you can discuss things.
- Be open to varied possibilities. Consider and evaluate relevant options before making decisions and choices.

This week I will explore my assumptions about aging and reimagine possibilities in ways I have not considered before.

CHAPTER 31

Too Much to Do: Managing
Life's Juggling Act

Do you ever feel like you're juggling too many balls in the air at the same time? Our lives are filled with responsibilities, challenges, and struggles. Sometimes, life's commotions and demands can have a positive impact, motivating us toward more optimal performance and action. Yet at other times, stress and the many facets of life's juggling act—meeting a deadline, anticipating a transition, balancing childcare or eldercare—can interfere with how we feel, how we live our day-to-day, and how we sleep at night.

In today's hectic, changing world, we experience stress on many fronts, such as relationships, health matters, work-life balance, transitions, losses, finances, and concern about current events and the environment (American Psychological Association, 2024). On a daily basis, let's face it, lots of us feel that we are focusing our attention and energies in too many places, with all of our have-to's, want-to's, responsibilities, and challenges. We may feel overwhelmed, fearing that at any moment we may lose our precarious sense of balance and the juggling act could come tumbling down.

Tumult, multiple demands, and worry can keep us from thinking clearly and cause us to be reactive, rather than planful. Neuroscience research reveals that our experiences change our brains. New thoughts and behaviors produce new pathways in the brain (Siegel, 2012). Thus, training our brains to focus our attention differently can generate alternate routes and responses in the brain. Taking quiet moments to get back on track can empower us to feel less caught up in imbalance and overwhelm. Instead, we can learn to pause, reflect, sift through ough possibilities, and choose more effective actions and behaviors.

Inspirations

You can transition toward regaining your balance with these six practices.

1 - How satisfied are you with the components of your life? Given your goals, responsibilities, and challenges, how can you move toward greater balance, fulfillment, productivity, and well-being?

Robert Biswas-Diener and Ben Dean identify ten pillars of a balanced life (Biswas-Diener & Dean, 2007). These include profession, finance, physical environment, spirituality, intimacy, family, social support, home/ office, fun/play, growth and learning, and overall satisfaction in life.

You can take a look at these ten domains in your own life and work. Write them across the top of a piece of paper. Then, ask yourself what you have been doing and where you see yourself (Biswas-Diener & Dean, 2007). Consider each domain, one at a time. Then, using a scale from one to ten, identify your satisfaction level. Write a word or sentence summarizing your level of satisfaction in each area. Which pillar is calling for your attention? In which pillar could even a small change improve your sense of well-being and reduce your experience of overwhelm and stress?

2 – What's most important to you? Invite yourself to reflect on your priorities. Sometimes, everything seems important. The to-do list can feel endless, containing tasks that you need to do, want to do, or others want us to do (Berns-Zare, 2020d).

Meet Emma. Emma realized that her level of satisfaction with fun and play in her life was quite low. She gave this area a 4 on her *Pillars of a Balanced Life*. As she reflected, she felt that she was either working at her job or taking care of family responsibilities most of the time. Emma decided to raise her self-assessment for fun/play to a 5 in the next 30 days by taking three hours each week just for herself to take care of her own wants and needs, such as a manicure, a run at the park, or dinner with a dear friend. Emma's action plan: On her calendar each week she created an appointment with herself called "Emma's Joyful Moments." She typed it in bright blue ink. For example: *Emma's Joyful Moments – Dinner with BFF ☺ Thursday 6:00-9:00 pm.*

Have you been neglecting an important aspect of your life? What would it take to nudge this area just a bit higher in your satisfaction level? What small shift can you make in your priorities in the next 30 days to help you get there?

Here are a few questions to help you reflect on your priorities:

- What do I feel is the best use of my time [today, this week, this month]?
- Which tasks or activities may bring me closer to the outcomes I desire?
- Which tasks or activities may help me strengthen my relationships and connections?
- If left undone, which actions or inactions may have significant negative consequences, and which will not?

Take a few moments daily or weekly to pause, listen to your inner voice, reflect, and discern. Consider your priorities. You might choose to reorganize them with your new awareness and record them in your journal, notebook or electronic device. Then, at intervals, perhaps weekly, evaluate how you're doing and choose your next step or steps.

3 - Remind yourself to have realistic expectations. Unrealistic expectations may cause feelings of overwhelm, stress, and exhaustion and may compromise your wellbeing and effectiveness. Offer yourself calm, patience, and perspective as you create change.

You might look at your to-do lists, pause, and ask yourself a few questions, such as:

- What can I realistically expect from myself given that I (like everyone else) have only 24 hours each day?
- Will this task make a difference in a week, a month, or a year?

- Given my priorities, what's important now? What can wait? What can I delete or ask someone else to do?
- Is there a less extensive expectation or goal that would meet this need or want and still satisfy me?
- How can I accomplish this goal, even if it takes a while? For example: *I'll clean out the storage area in stages. I'll take one class each semester, rather than two or volunteer once a week, rather than twice a week.*

4 – Ask for help. What resources might assist you? Instead of trying to do everything yourself, can you ask for some help? You might be surprised at what people are willing to offer. Ask for help, experience the sense of relief, and share your gratitude for the assistance.

5 – Find rest in contemplative or mindful moments. Pausing to mindfully notice your intuitions, emotions, and feelings, and cultivating contemplative or spiritual practices can enrich your experience and reduce feelings of overwhelm. What practices might help you open some space within yourself? Take a moment to rest and reflect.

6 – Practice Gratitude. Acknowledging the goodness in your life can help you shift from feelings of being overwhelmed to more positive emotions (Emmons & McCullough, 2003; Seligman et al., 2005).

Try this: Think of 1-2 things that went well today. Reflect on what you are grateful for or what went right. It can help to be specific as you consider and record these gratitudes.

This week I'll let my feelings of overwhelm remind me to pause for quiet moments of reflection and discernment, choose my priorities, and set realistic expectations.

CHAPTER 32

The Wisdom of
Simplicity -- Kindergarten and Life

A few years ago, I was a guest reader in the kindergarten class of my 6-year-old grandson. It was a joy to share a favorite book with my guy, his classmates, and their wonderful teacher. Although my chief objective was to help the children with their learning, it turned out that the children taught me a few lessons too (Berns-Zare, 2019).

Let me share some experiences. The children all sat on a large, colorful floormat facing me with my grandson on one side. While I read aloud, one student became quietly upset because another child had taken his place on the mat. When the youngster told the teacher, she simply and wisely asked the two of them, "How can you fix this?" The pair talked for a moment. Then one child moved over slightly, and the two shared the space. The argument was quickly resolved, and the boys returned to listening to the story.

The kindergartners listened quietly and attentively as we shared the story. When I asked questions, most raised their hands, waiting patiently for their turns. When a child forgot and spoke out of turn, another child would remind them to raise their hand. Most of the time, the children listened to the suggestions of their peers, providing many young learners with opportunities to speak, be heard, and make good decisions.

Overall, the children took care of the business of being good classroom citizens. They were practicing their emerging social-emotional intelligence skills as they interacted in the classroom (Elias, 2006; 1999; Goleman, 1995). They demonstrated awareness of their own feelings and the feelings of others as they interacted with kindness and empathy and made responsible decisions regarding their behavior. When I accidentally turned two pages instead of one, my beloved, alert six-year-old grandson quietly stood up and in a polite, hushed voice showed me the page I had missed. When I finished reading, some children said thank you. And, later during a science activity, I spotted one kindergartner kindly assisting a classmate who was struggling to accomplish her tasks.

Consider the wisdom, generosity, and resilience of this young microcosm of humanity. Respecting each individual's differing needs and abilities. Solving problems and helping each other. Sitting quietly and listening. Laughing together. Arguing over territory and fixing the disagreement by peacefully moving aside to create space. Sharing kindness and gratitude.

Some years ago, author Rob Fulghum (1986) wrote that many of life's important lessons can be learned in kindergarten. Could some of life's solutions really be that simple?

Inspirations

This week you might experiment with one of these inspirational strategies.

- Notice personal character strengths and positive behaviors in children and adolescents (Waters, 2017). When you spot a youngster's strength or see them doing something right, call it as you see it. For example, if your nephew or niece offers you assistance carrying groceries, you might say "Thank you for being so observant and kind to help me carry these heavy bags." During a discussion, you might comment, "I noticed how you were listening so carefully when [---] was speaking. I'll bet they really appreciated your kind attention."

- Consider the questions: "What can I learn from the wisdom of youth?" and "What can they learn from me?"

- What two or three significant lessons have you learned during your lifetime that you might want to share with a young person? How could you offer these teachings to a child or teenager in your life or community?

**This week I will think about some of
the simple, yet powerful lessons I learned,
or wish I'd learned, in my youth.**

CHAPTER 33

Love of Learning in this
Season of Your Life

Along my own path, I find that no matter what my age or season of life, my essential self continues to flow with the rhythms of the academic calendar. Inspired by spring's late blossoms, I am drawn toward both the closure of the rigors of the school year: the fall, winter, and early spring, and the emergence of new growth in the natural world. Then, as one who loves learning, I look forward to a peaceful summer pause to slow down, catch up, read, visualize, and plan for the months ahead. When the midwestern summer bursts forth with color and warmth, I am drawn toward contemplation, rest and renewal. As I observe nature's rhythms turning to autumn, I find myself ready to generate next steps, eager to dive into new learnings, skills and adventures. My inner "forever student" continues to circle back within these seasonal cycles in each phase of my life.

Perhaps it's no surprise that love of learning is one of my top character strengths. I think of myself as a life-long learner. While I may not master everything I study, I treasure experiences of learning and growing.

Where does learning fit in *your* life? Whether love of learning is one of your top strengths or a strength you want or need to build on, continuing to learn and sharing what you learn with others can offer greater joy, understanding and meaning in your life (Niemiec, 2017).

Learning new skills, deepening insights, gaining knowledge or other kinds of growth activities can be accomplished in formal atmospheres like schools or training programs and also informally in the contexts of life, leisure, and work. Not only is a thirst for knowledge and expanding one's understandings linked with academic achievement, these strengths can also enhance positive experiences and wellbeing (Niemiec, 2017).

The ability to learn is enhanced by a growth mindset (Dweck, 2006). Mindset, as discussed in Chapter 8, conceptualizes the brain as a muscle you can develop. Choosing to exercise a growth mindset can lead you toward greater skill development, enhanced understandings, and transformation, reminding you that with effort and perseverance you can indeed learn and grow.

Any decade in which you find yourself can offer opportunities to learn and to journey beyond your certainties toward greater understandings and personal development. While sometimes the focus of learning is simply to take in new information, learning can also transform your perceptions and discernments about yourself and this world, impacting your roles, choices, and actions. As you learn, you can connect more greatly not only to topics and information but also to contemporary understandings, new concepts,, and future generations of learners and teachers.

Inspirations

Here are a few ideas to help you empower yourself as a life-long learner. You may want to write about your experiences and gleanings in your journal, notebook, or in notes on your electronic device.

Remember that you can learn, not only from successes but also from setbacks and failures. As you learn and grow, keep in mind that any experience can offer opportunities for learning or to view or do things differently next time.

- Set a goal to learn something new each day, such as a fact, quote, skill, or strategy. For example: You might learn how to water an indoor plant correctly, how to hang a picture on the wall of your living space, or how to repair something. You might experiment with a skill such as using the computer mouse with your non-dominant hand, throwing a football, preparing a new recipe, experimenting with a new language, or trying yoga or a new leadership skill. You might investigate a topic of interest, view an informational video, or explore a saying or quote that feels meaningful.

- Engage your curiosity to learn something new about a topic you're interested in. Search the internet, have a conversation with an expert, read a book about it, or listen to a podcast.
- Realize that learning and growth can take time. You may find it useful to learn step-by-step, letting yourself appreciate that layers of information and skills that are unfamiliar or difficult can accumulate one piece at a time. It can be helpful to scaffold your learning and practice in smaller steps or chunks (Stanford University, 2025).
- Ask a youth, peer, or older adult to share a bit of wisdom with you or teach you something (even for a moment or two). You may be surprised by what you learn, and you may bring a few moments of meaning into that person's life.
- Partner with a friend to learn. Choose something you want to learn or a skill to develop. Partner with your friend to set objectives, accountabilities, and move forward toward your desired outcomes. If you get stuck, ask your friend to help you work around the obstacle.

What new concepts or insights can you bring into your life?

This week I will consider the role of learning in my life and take at least a few moments to learn something new.

CHAPTER 34

Practicing Gratitude

Where does gratitude fit in your everyday life? How often do you pause to appreciate pleasant moments, gifts, and other good stuff? A key element of a life well-lived, gratitude acknowledges that we've experienced something of value, whether tangible or intangible. A grateful mindset can shift how we view our experiences, opening ourselves to thankfulness and noticing positives and goodness, rather than looking away or taking them for granted.

Although we hear a lot about gratitude these days, it's not a new practice. Recognized in ancient spiritual teachings and writings, in today's world the benefits of gratitude are well validated in social science research. Mounting evidence associates gratitude with enhanced feelings of personal wellbeing, self-esteem, creativity, and happiness (Emmons, 2007; 2016; Emmons & Mishra, 2012). Practicing gratitude can improve your connections with others, boosting the wellbeing of giver and receiver. Thankfulness can help us feel more energized, expand our levels of life satisfaction, and bolster wellbeing during difficult times.

According to University of California psychologist Robert Emmons, gratitude is more than a simple feeling. It involves acknowledging that someone or something has brought goodness into our lives, inviting us to view some experiences as gifts. While it may not come easily to some of us, thankfulness is a readily accessible skill that we can learn and get better at. Emmons recommends cultivating gratitude as an ongoing practice in our day-to-day lives to foster happiness and wellbeing .

Inspirations

Life offers many opportunities to pay attention to circumstances, events, and relationships that motivate thankfulness. And there are many ways to practice gratitude. Here are a few practices.

- **Developing a routine gratitude practice.** Each day write down a few things you are thankful for. Your journal or notebook is a good place to write, or you might create a gratitude space on your electronic device. Focus on what's going *right*. It can be as simple as recalling a person who acknowledged or helped you, something you experienced, or a meaningful moment.

- **Writing a letter of gratitude and sharing it.** Think about someone who has changed your life in an important way (Seligman, 2011). Write a letter to that person. You might explain in detail how that person helped you and thank them for the kindness. Be specific as you comment about the difference they made in your life. Then call or email that person. If appropriate, ask if you can visit and don't say why. Show up and read your letter.

- **Doing something helpful.** Even the smallest gestures can make a positive difference to you and the person you share it with. Open a door for someone, donate or volunteer at the local food pantry, share your time, invite someone to get in front of you in line, or do a random act of kindness.

- **Noticing the gift of your breath.** Pause and take a mindful moment to inhale and exhale. Invite yourself to notice with awe or radical amazement the fact that you are breathing. Or simply pay attention to the sensation of breath as it flows in and out.

***This week I will choose a way
to practice gratitude each day.***

CHAPTER 35

Where Are You Right Now?

Life is filled with distractions. It's common to fall into the habit of mindlessly doing, checking things off lists that may not be integral to our values, who we are, or what is important. Sometimes, our thoughts wander to what's next, anticipating moments, hours, days, years that have not yet happened. Without creating "breathing space," we may find ourselves preoccupied, drifting, or overwhelmed, rather than present and balanced.

Where are *you* right now, in this moment? Do you ever find yourself physically present, but so distracted that you have no idea what's going on right here, right now?

When was the last time you intentionally paused to simply notice *now*? This kind of paying attention, resting your awareness and attention on where you are in the present moment, is the definition of mindfulness. And research reveals the many benefits of mindfulness, including connections between mindfulness and health, well-being, and positive emotions (Goleman & Davidson, 2017). Jon Kabat-Zinn, founder of the Center for Mindfulness at the University of Massachusetts Medical School, writes that although we can get lost in our possibilities, the reality is that the current moment is all we really have (1994). Our lives reveal themselves moment by moment.

Mindfulness is often explained as intentionally paying attention to the present moment with a non-judgmental attitude. That is, noticing our personal here-and-now experience, and rather than getting swept away by it, letting it go without negativity, judgement, or criticism (Kabat-Zinn, 1994, 2012; Siegel, 2011). In mindfulness practice, as we notice whatever thoughts that arise, we can simply release them, returning to a focus on our breath or other anchor.

Mindfulness is not just a nice idea or a one-time fix we perform once and then own. More accurately, like practicing piano keyboarding or reading skills, mindfulness requires cultivation and practice. We learn to notice our thoughts or sensations as they arise and then let them go. Perhaps we set an intention to pay attention to our breathing. We breathe, the mind wanders, we return our attention to the breath, and again the mind wanders. During just a few moments of mindfulness practice, this wandering away and then returning may occur many times. When the mind wanders, we can gently let our intention toward mindfulness simply call us back to this present moment.

Meditation researchers Jon Kabat-Zinn and Richard Davidson asked participants working at a biotech startup company to use the Mindfulness Based Stress Reduction program daily for 30 minutes during an 8-week period (Goleman & Davidson, 2017; Williams & Penman, 2011). Their findings showed remarkable changes in areas of the brain related to positive emotions and energy. And mindfulness is one of the key components for building self-compassion (Warren et al., 2016). Self-compassion, regarding ourselves with care, emotional safety, and kindness in challenging situations, can help us become aware of our experiences in a balanced way, recognizing our thoughts and emotions, while not exaggerating them. As we practice mindful self-compassion, we can strengthen our emotional resilience, learning to lessen the hold of negative emotions and inviting more positive emotions of self-kindness.

Inspirations

Consider including mindfulness meditation in your second half of life toolbox. Practicing mindful attention can help you gently train the mind in positive ways, aiding concentration and the capacity to relate more effectively to what's happening right now. Mindfulness can be practiced for a moment, a few moments, or a longer time, helping you more intentionally focus your attention.

To practice mindfulness, locate yourself in a space where you feel safe and comfortable. Take a moment to pause what you're doing.

- Settle into a position that feels comfortable for you. Perhaps allow your eyes to close or lower in a softened gaze.
- Simply notice your breathing (or another focal point if you prefer) There's no need to change anything. Just invite your attention toward the natural rhythm of your own breath as it enters and leaves your body.
- When your mind wanders (which minds often do) to another moment, issue, or plan, just notice, and without judgment bring yourself back home to your breathing. Tenderly let wandering thoughts go as though they are quietly drifting away in a breeze.
- As often as needed, gently let yourself return to one breath, one breath, one breath.
- When you feel ready after a moment or a few moments, open your eyes with full alertness.

Mindfulness practice is handy, portable, and available when you gently call upon it. For example, I like to begin some meetings with a moment of mindfulness. At the start of the gathering, sometimes I suggest a brief pause for people, including myself, to turn attention to the breath, another anchor, or a repeated phrase to help focus and become present.

You don't have to be a yogi to benefit from mindfulness meditation. Just like learning to drive or to swim, mindfulness is a learnable skill. Where are *you* right now? How can you fold more mindful moments into the flow of your life? Go lightly and compassionately with yourself.

This week I will choose moments to pause, breathe, and practice mindfulness.

CHAPTER 36

Hope and Taking Action
Toward Your Goals

What do you hope for? Even during uncertain times, adversity, and life's transitions, hope can endure. Our hope may feel solid and sure, or it may ebb and flow amid life's shifts, events, and our own internal lenses.

During the COVID-19 pandemic I thought a lot about hope. In the precariousness of that period, I hoped most people affected would survive and recover. I hoped my life would rebound to a new normal in which I and most people could find a sense of comfort, balance, and forward momentum. I hoped I could soon be with loved ones, friends, and community.

I learned that hope is a choice we can make. From the work of Dr. Viktor Frankl, we learn that we always have a choice, that emotional health is influenced by the attitudes we choose, the decisions we make, and the ability to look forward rather than backward (1959; 1985).

Hope involves an understanding that we have the capacity, pathways, and resolve to reach toward our goals (Snyder, 2000; Snyder, et al., 2002). But hope is more than simply understanding or belief. Hope involves a positive attitude and positive actions. Thus, actionable hope is not simply wishful thinking. Rather hope involves taking initiative and implementing our goals with intentionally goal-oriented motivation and action (Feldman & Dreher, 2011).

According to hope theory, developed by C.R. Snyder, hope is goal-centered and includes three components: (1) a goal; (2) agency, which involves the motivation, determination, and attitude that the goal can be achieved; and (3) pathways, steps toward our goal and backup plans to reach it if one of our steps doesn't work. Hope has been associated with emotional wellbeing, personal growth goals, academic and athletic achievement (Cheavens, et al., 2019; Feldman, et al., 2019; Snyder, et al., 2002).

Inspirations

These four steps can help you guide yourself toward greater hope, resolve, and action.

1 – **Choose a Goal.** Whether short-term or long-term, small or large, having a goal offers direction and a pathway to help you steer yourself forward. A goal that is clear, specific and positive is likely to be more effective than a vague, general goal.

2 – **Create a workable pathway toward your goal.** Generate multiple routes or strategies to lead you toward your desired goal, including alternatives if the first route doesn't get you there successfully. What are your options? What else might you try if needed?

3 – **Engage your sense of agency or self-efficacy.** Continue to motivate yourself. Bolster yourself with affirming messages that boost your confidence, perseverance, and motivation to continue toward your desired goal, even when you confront obstacles and roadblocks. Examples of hopeful self-talk: "I can work my way through this," and "I'll keep trying despite the obstacles."

4 – **Visualize yourself reaching your goal.** Pause daily and imagine yourself actually achieving your goal (Feldman & Dreher, 2011). Invite yourself to imagine the thoughts and feelings you experience as you reach your objective and live your new reality.

This week I will activate hope in my life with a clear goal, actions to steer me toward my destination and alternatives in case I need them. Then, I'll motivate myself with positive self-talk and visualize myself reaching my goal.

CHAPTER 37

Quieting the Inner Critic
with Self-Compassion

All of us make mistakes, misjudgments, missteps. Personal foibles are part of being human.

Are you sometimes confronted with self-doubts? Do you have nagging thoughts that you're not good enough? You're not alone. Private self-bullying conversations are common to many of us as we navigate our lives. Often called the "inner critic," this negative, self-critical voice can undermine how we feel about ourselves, our goals, and our effectiveness. Conquering the inner critic can help you create a kinder, more productive relationship with yourself.

According to self-compassion researcher Kristin Neff, the antidote for self-criticism and harsh self-judgment is self-compassion. Self-compassion is treating ourselves kindly. Accepting our strengths and our imperfections and offering ourselves the same goodwill we would share with someone we care about.

Evidence indicates that self-compassion is not only good for our wellbeing but also a more effective motivator than fear (Neff, 2011). Self-compassion can quiet the inner critic, opening the doors to greater confidence and feelings of security. This acceptance and love guided inward boosts our body's capacity to produce oxytocin, a hormone that influences our social interaction and emotional bonding. Conversely, fear provokes feelings of insecurity and self-doubt, putting our brains and bodies on alert and triggering the fight-or-flight stress reaction.

Research reveals that self-compassion is not just a soft, feel-good choice. Rather, it can actually strengthen our ability to cope with transitions and challenging situations, such as setbacks, disappointments, illness, divorce, loss of job, and retirement. Self-kindness can also lead us to engage in healthier life-style behaviors, such as nutritional eating and exercise (Neff, 2011; Neff & Germer, 2019). In short, self-compassion can help us feel happier and function more effectively.

Inspirations

Here are six inspirations to help you quiet self-criticism and create a kinder, more compassionate relationship with yourself.

1 – **Notice what you're thinking about.** Acknowledge your self-critical thoughts when they occur. Then remind yourself that the inner critic voice is only a thought—that just because you're thinking about something, it is *not* necessarily true. Remind yourself that thoughts and attitudes can be inaccurate, exaggerated, and biased by your personal emotions and experiences. And that it's possible to reframe or modify your thoughts.

2 - **Respond to the inner critic by replacing negative critical thoughts with more accurate, positive information.** When you notice yourself repeating a harsh thought about yourself, you can choose self-affirmation with kinder self-talk.

For example, a thought such as "I make too many mistakes, I'll never reach my goal" can be balanced with a statement such as "I can learn and grow from my mistakes, and each one is another step toward reaching my goal." Try writing down your repetitive inner critic thoughts and then generating alternative positive statements you want to replace them with.

3 – **Release the inner critic.** When you notice that critical inner voice, invite yourself to release it, let it go, or put it aside. For example, if you're working on a project or assignment and thinking a self-critical

thought, you might toss this criticism in the garbage can or throw it in a jar and tightly close the lid. This strategy can offer a recess so you can move forward toward completing the task.

4 – **Embrace imperfection with self-compassion**. Imperfection is simply part of the human condition. When we are being too hard on ourselves, self-compassion, kindness channeled inward toward ourselves, offers balance and a healing intention to reduce needless suffering. Neff and Germer (2019) suggest that rather than resist our internal bullying, we can accept that life is difficult, that we are all imperfect humans living imperfect existences.

Try this practice when you want to quiet the inner critic:

- Pause.
- Gently ask yourself these questions: "How do I feel?" and "What do I need now?"
- Grant yourself a moment of warm-hearted self-compassion. Simply acknowledge that you are where you are, even if you don't know the answer or how to respond to your needs or the situation right now.
- You might want to rest your hand softly at your heart space as you offer yourself kindness in the moment.

5 – **Remember you are part of our interconnected world**. Check in with a supportive friend, colleague, or family member when your inner critic is shouting and you need a boost. Discuss the situation, request a reality check and some cheerleading. Have a "shortlist" of people you trust and can count on to offer you encouragement, common sense, and compassion when you need it.

6 – **Each day be kind to yourself with self-care.** Can you offer yourself a few minutes to take care of your mind, body, spirit? For example, take a walk, listen to your favorite music, go for a swim or bike ride, enjoy the sunset, play with a pet, do some yoga, engage in mindfulness practice, or do something else you enjoy.

This week I will be kinder to myself, overcoming self-doubts with self-compassion.

CHAPTER 38

Navigating toward Greater
Equanimity in Your Life

Today's culture prizes doing, accomplishing, action, and more, more, more. If we buy into this relentless busyness, we may miss out on quiet moments that can offer us essential nourishment and renewal of mind, body, and spirit.

Many of us crave greater balance in our lives. In the persistent challenges of our day-to-day, we may lose our balance among the calm waters, moderate waves, and turbulent storms we encounter. Although steadiness may seem elusive, we can seek gentler rhythms of rest and activity, play and work, inhale and exhale that offer moments of joy, tranquility, and rest.

Lately, I've been thinking about the practice of *equanimity*. I'm aware of how easily stirred I sometimes feel when I get caught up in the precarious whims of life's heavy winds. Equanimity honors the wisdom of balance as we ride the waves of life. Yet, this kind of balance does *not* require us to retreat from our activities, responsibilities, or work. Rather, equanimity is a capacity for even-mindedness and steadiness despite the situations we find ourselves in. It is a calm power of observation that enables us to be present without becoming overly caught up in what we see and experience. Like a sailboat that remains upright even in heavy storms, equanimity helps the sails sway in the breezes, holding centeredness, rather than being pulled too far in any direction for too long.

Well-developed equanimity invites a capacity for inner steadfastness, an ability to remain upright in stormy times. Like exercising, eating healthier foods, or meditation, equanimity can be cultivated through habit and practice. We can set an intention to navigate toward the internal spaciousness that equanimity offers. Then, we practice. Gradually, we can develop quieting habits of mind, learning to reclaim moments of greater composure and refuge, more calmly adjusting our emotions and responses amid the dramatic winds of our lives.

Inspirations

Here are a few strategies to help you navigate toward greater equanimity and balance in your life.

Understand that equanimity is *not* indifference or passivity. As you practice equanimity you can empower yourself to face life's struggles and challenges, acknowledging the realities of a situation, while not being pulled emotionally too far in any direction. You might draw on a strength, such as perspective, self-regulation, or spirituality to help you regain balance and centeredness, as you deal with the challenges you encounter. And when you find that you've been tugged further emotionally than you'd like, cultivating equanimity can help you return to a more centered way of being present.

From this vantage point, it's possible to respond calmly, with resolve and action. Equanimity can assist you in your personal and professional life, as well as when engaging wrongs, oppression, and other issues that confront you in your communities and your world.

Invite yourself to to begin from where you are today. Twenty-first century life presents many challenges. For example, increasing demands of work, life transitions, health issues, losses, and social struggles. We may yearn for the way things were before a change or feel upset about the way things are, but these habitual thought patterns and emotions can impede calm, acceptance and action.

Consider adopting a "this too shall pass" attitude, an understanding that changes, transitions, and obstacles are expectable realities of life. Cultivating evenness, calmness, and self-compassion can lead to acceptance that you are enough, that you can adjust your responses, and that it's okay to begin where you are today.

Strengthen equanimity with mindful presence. Mindfulness practice offers opportunities to observe life's ebbs and flows with a sense of inner balance and spaciousness. Of course, we lose our balance, but then how do we return to greater equanimity? Keep in mind that mindfulness is much more about how you relate to what's happening than about the event itself (Salzberg, 2024). Thus, practicing greater equanimity invites you toward liberation beyond the stories you tell yourself, reclaiming your attention and well-being in the realities of the present moment.

Even when it feels that stormy weather is pulling you in unwanted directions, the gentle discipline of returning to greater calm and balance in the moment is a powerful act of compassion for yourself.

To experiment with mindful equanimity, take a pause and breathe. Invite yourself toward quiet and calm. Rather than fighting with the challenge or situation, consider how you might notice it with less judgment, offering yourself space to simply observe what's happening.

Gently rest your awareness on your breath or other focal point. As your mind wanders, invite yourself to gently return to the rhythms of your breath as you reclaim the present moment. You can return repeatedly to the flow of your breathing. Experience the peace of greater equanimity and calm in the present moment.

For more ideas on practicing mindfulness, refer to Chapters 7, 13, and 29 in this book.

This week I will empower myself as I navigate toward greater equanimity and balance, one moment at a time.

CHAPTER 39

Starting Whether
You Like It or Not

"I know I should do this, but I don't feel like doing it." "I don't have time, there's too much going on." "I wish I could get started, but ..."

Do these refrains of procrastination sound familiar? Unfortunately, for many of us, this melody never seems to get old. Like a familiar ballad filled with longing, thoughts like these may too often recall where we *wish* we were but don't seem able to get to.

Procrastination is simply putting things off. We all procrastinate sometimes. But let's face it, some of us put things off more than others. According to Joseph Ferrari, professor of psychology at DePaul University, about 20 percent of people in the United States are chronic procrastinators (American Psychological Association, 2010). Ferrari explains that procrastination is not just delaying but purposely waiting to decide or act.

Speaking for myself, although not typically a procrastinator, I do have places where I get stuck in non-doing and waiting to act. The sad song I've been singing involves organizing family photos. There are many, many photos sitting in boxes stored at my home. We have more boxes of photos than I'd like to count. My family has taken many photos, while others are inherited from loved ones. Too many pictures! Well, we still have most of them, and I need to get started on this formidable task.

Is it worth taking a second look at something *you* have avoided starting? For some folks, occasional avoidance of a task is not much of a problem.

For others, procrastination is unwanted habitual behavior. For example, Carla hopes to earn a promotion at work. She's had four weeks to complete an important project. A busy manager, she gets distracted "putting out fires" with her team (Berns-Zare, 2018). Each day, she says she'll start the project, yet each day she avoids starting. Now the project is due in two days. Telling herself she works better under pressure, Carla works late the night before it's due. Realizing she could have done a better job if she'd started earlier, she's mad at herself for habitually putting things off. Does Carla's story sound familiar?

Inspirations

According to procrastination expert, Timothy Pychyl, the first step to change the procrastination habit is becoming aware of your patterns (2021). Making a list of typically delayed tasks and the thoughts and feelings involved can be a good place to begin. You may want to use your notebook, journal, or electronic device.

Here are ten tips to help you (and me) move forward with our goals:

Begin the task with the conclusion in mind. Define your goal. Be specific and state it clearly. What would you like to have accomplished when the project is completed? How do you feel about your goal, and how do you want to feel? Remember that you have the freedom to choose what you do, how you do it, and are responsible for your choices. You might want to write down your goal and post it where you can see it daily.

Just get started. Even minimal progress toward your goal can help you feel more positive about the objective and yourself (Sheldon, 2004). Once you begin the task, you may discover it's not as "bad" as you'd anticipated.

Begin somewhere! Take one small step. Then another, then another to get the ball rolling down the hill toward completion. The great Chinese philosopher Lao Tzu is known to have said "A journey of a thousand miles begins with one step."

For example, Mark needs to file his income tax return. He's been avoiding it. Finally, he takes the first step.

- Day 1: He creates a file and looks for his receipts and other documents. He congratulates himself for getting started.
- Day 2: He starts organizing the documents and looks through his bank statements. The momentum stimulates his motivation to move forward.
- Day 3: He fills out the tax information form provided by his accountant.
- Day 4: He finishes organizing his materials.
- Day 5: He makes an appointment with his accountant.
- Day 6: He completes his preparation and meets with his accountant.
- Day 7: Feeling a sense of relief, he signs and releases his forms.

Be Prepared – Create an If-Then Plan. Think ahead to form contingency plans if needed when the going gets tough (Legrand et al., 2017; Oettingen, 2017; 2024). An if-then plan can help you overcome "I can't" and "I don't want to."

For example:

> "If I want to check my email during the hour, then I'll turn my phone off and continue doing my task."
> "If I feel bored when I'm doing this task, then I'll take a breath, focus my attention, and keep working."
> "If I feel like I need to eat a sugary snack, then I will walk for ten minutes instead."

Remember You Don't Have to Like It to Do It. To achieve a goal, your current level of motivation does *not* have to be high. You can carry out a task even when you don't feel ready or motivated to do it (Pychl, 2010). Just beginning the task can positively shift your motivation and attitude.

Engage your growth mindset. Adopting a growth mindset can bring us optimistic ways to face challenges, get started, and persevere toward goals (Dweck, 2006). The belief that you can improve and that your abilities will blossom with effort and hard work can strengthen the capacity to accomplish your objectives.

- Speak to yourself from a growth mindset perspective, such as: *"Lots of successful people have a tough time getting started or struggle along the way. I can take that first step and deal with whatever challenges arise."*
- Remember that you have choices. How do you interpret failures and challenges along the way? How can you shift toward more positive, affirming self-talk to help you move toward accomplishing your goal?

Plan Realistically. It's helpful to get a practical understanding of what's needed to complete the task effectively and on time (Brown University, 2008).

- Break the task into small, manageable steps. Be honest about what you can do in a particular time frame.
- Allow yourself relaxation and reasonable rewards as you complete the steps.
- Keep track of your progress. Adjust tasks and your commitments as needed.
- Avoid perfectionism. Be reasonable about expectations of yourself, others, and the situation.

Consider available resources. Who can help you get this done: a family member, friend, consultant or coach? Discuss approaches, strategies, and options. Is there a skill you can learn or strengthen to help you accomplish this goal?

Rest and renew. Remember to take care of yourself. Get enough sleep, eat healthy foods, exercise in a way that respects your body and your abilities, interact with other people that you enjoy.

This week I will focus on a task I've been avoiding and get started, one step at a time.

CHAPTER 40

The Remarkable Power of Habit

I've been thinking about the importance of habits and their role in navigating our daily choices. Even when we're not aware of it, our habits, big and small, are the building blocks of our day-to-day behaviors. We open our eyes in the morning, get out of bed, brush our teeth, wash our faces. Most of us have routines for how we eat, engage with others, and deal with routine responsibilities.

To be honest, no one has been more awakened by these realizations than I have. Although I coach people on strategies for building habits, I personally have rebelled against the concept of habits, thinking of them as somewhat rigid and mundane. Now I understand that we all have habits, although some may be so automatic that we are unaware of them. In fact, many habits are fundamental in our lives, helping us conserve energy and live with greater efficiency, such as how we approach beginning our day or take care of the vehicle we drive. With these understandings, we can harness the habits we choose so that we can live our lives in ways that help us thrive.

Neuroscience shows that when we change our habits and try new experiences, we also change connections in our brains. Through a process called neuroplasticity, practicing and repeating habits can remodel areas of our brains. This happens as the brain produces new neural connections and strengthens existing pathways when we focus our attention, learn, and gain new skills and experiences (Siegel, 2011; 2012). Research reveals that brain development can continue throughout our lives. Even as we age, whether 50, 60, 70, 80 years old or beyond, when we develop and expand our habits, our brains grow new neural connections.

Greater awareness of our habits, the ones we like and the ones we'd like to change, can inform how we show up in our lives. With this awareness and a few strategic guideposts, we can make choices to maintain the habits that serve us well and change those that don't.

If we want to modify a habit or learn a new one, we can gain remarkable results by making one tiny change at time. In the beginning of developing a new habit, whether we want to change a "bad" habit or form a new one, creating the new habit can be more critical than achieving the goal. Transitions toward change are usually more effective when we begin gradually. Even getting just 1% better each day can help us create new habits (Hays, 2002; 2018).

Accumulating habits involves deciding the kind of person you want to be and then empowering your vision with a process of small wins emerging from habits (Clear, 2018). One step at a time, we can create our personal practices as these habits inform our way of learning, doing, and being in the world.

Inspirations

1 – **Start by building awareness.** Pay attention to your current habits and identify one habit you want to change in some way. Notice your typical procedures step by step. It can help to simply make a list of your daily routines and steps (Berns-Zare, 2020d).

2 – **Change begins with making a choice.** What habits do you like? For example, you enjoy your morning coffee with sugar, but don't like the fact that you eat two sweet rolls with it and have been gaining weight. Which habit(s) are you willing to take steps to change?

3 - **Attach a new habit or behavior to something you already do regularly.** One strategy, called *habit stacking* connects a new habit with a long-established habit (Clear, 2018). For example: to add a moment of

mindfulness to your routine, you might create this time right after you brush your teeth each morning. *After I brush my teeth, I will sit down and breathe mindfully for two minutes.* If you want to begin walking daily, you might plan to take your walk for 20 minutes right after lunch or before dinner.

4 – **Gain greater clarity about what you want to do and how you will do it.** Be specific and bite off just a small chunk at a time. Research suggests the efficacy of beginning with a specific implementation intention or *if-then* plan: *If* I'm in this situation, *then* I'll do this (Oettingen & Gollwitzer, 2010). For example: *If it's 12 noon, then I'll stop what I'm doing and walk for two minutes.*

5 – **Keep the change simple and strengthen it with repetition and consistency.** Let yourself know that one small step at a time can add up to powerful new habits and behaviors. James Clear (2018) recommends "the two minute rule" as you begin a new habit or behavior -- Break the habit into a small enough chunk that it can be accomplished in two minutes or less. For example, if you want to begin to lift weights or do yoga, start your practice with just a two-minute window: *After my shower each evening, I'll get on my yoga mat (or lift weights) for two minutes.* Or if you want to start practicing mindfulness meditation: *When I wake up each morning, I'll practice mindfulness for two minutes before I get out of bed.*

6 – **Remember the "*why.*"** Keeping in mind *why* we're doing something, the personal value, meaning, and importance of a behavior can be very helpful. According to performance psychologist Kate Hays, during practice and performance it is pivotal to remember your purpose, returning to your very personal reasons about why this is important to you. Dr. Hays notes the advantages of working toward being excellent rather than perfect (2018). This can apply to simple and more complex behavior changes.

This week I will pay attention to my habits and choose to change one, taking one small step at a time.

CHAPTER 41

Performing at Your Best in Life and Work

At various points in our lives, we are called to perform. Maybe we are interviewing for a job or volunteer position, speaking at a community meeting or family event, competing in a 5K run/walk, giving a presentation at work, auditioning for a local musical group, or improving our health after an injury or illness. If we're not prepared, the pressures we experience may get the best of us, blocking our capacity to perform and be present to the best of our ability.

When facing a challenge, it helps to be aware of the amount of pressure we're experiencing in our minds and bodies. Some tension can be helpful, but not too much. It's important to know what the optimal amount of tension is for us as individuals, the stress level at which we perform at our best. This involves awareness of what we want to be feeling, thinking, and experiencing in *this* situation. According to performance expert Kate Hays (2018), it's not helpful to be too anxious but also not to be too calm if we want to have optimal energy for our performance.

One way to manage our level of tension is diaphragmatic breathing. Sometimes called belly breathing, this strategy involves inhaling and exhaling fully to create space for oxygen and help direct focus and concentration. Improving performance can start with mindful breathing, training ourselves to systematically return to awareness of the breath as a tactic to clear the mind and bring greater focus. Practicing mindful breathing can also have important physical and psychological benefits.

Sometimes, we're not at 100% full power. One option in these situations is to respond with our 80% edge. Rather than thinking about what we can't do, we can strive to give 100% of the 80% available. Although it would be great to always be at 100%, this may not be possible. According to Dr. Hays, maybe today you're at 80% of your capacity to perform, but then what you may want to do is give 100% of that 80% (2017; 2018). This concept lets you be as fully present as possible, rather than giving all or nothing.

The 80% edge concept can empower you to be good enough in this moment, right here and now, even when you are not at your best or the situation is not ideal. This strategy invites you to allow yourself some self-compassion and self-forgiveness, which can be a good thing in performance situations.

Finally, remembering your "why" can provide a motivating force toward performing as you'd like to. Knowing why an activity is meaningful to you and why you are doing it, can remind you about the personal meaning, value, and importance of performing (Hays, 2018; Sinek, 2009). During practice and performance, at optimal moments, you can return your thoughts to why this situation matters to you. Not the external reasons, but your own personal reasons. That is, focusing on what is important about this to you is *not* a demand for perfection but can be a supportive motivator toward optimal performance.

Inspirations

- **Remember why you're doing it.** Whatever the performance or activity may be, you can tune into what it means to you, the "why." Remind yourself *why* this endeavor is important to you and let that knowledge support you as you approach your goal.
- **Remember to breathe during preparation and performance.** Mindful breath awareness (unless it feels uncomfortable to you)

can bolster your capacity to be present in the moment, bring oxygen into your body, and improve your focus.

- **Let yourself know you are enough.** Rather than striving for perfection, work toward excellence from where you are today, and try to give 100% of what you've got.

This week I will think about where I perform in life, tune into one area I'd like to improve, and empower myself toward change one step at a time.

CHAPTER 42

Leading with Supportive, Mindful Communication

How do you see yourself as a leader or role model in this season of your life?

There are many ways to lead. You may be a leader or role model in your family, community, workplace, or organization. Maybe you are simply the leader of your own life. Whatever leadership niche fits how you see yourself in this season of your life, how can you communicate mindfully and support your own interests, while also supporting and inspiring others?

However you see your leadership involvement, I want to offer the idea that our complex world benefits when leaders and role models are mindful and compassionate. Clearly, there are many kinds of leaders and role models in today's world, and each of us can choose to leverage our own capacity to lead in big and small ways throughout our lives, whether in our work, volunteer pursuits, or our personal activities. We can collaborate, build relationships, and participate in teams, task forces, or with families, friends, and community groups. Whatever our role, supportive mindful communication carries the potential to invigorate interactions and inspire positive outcomes, energy, relationship building, and engagement.

Positive leadership, formally and informally, can be enhanced by being attentively present in the moment. Leading mindfully can encourage the heart with authentic behaviors that show caring and appreciation for the values and spirits of others (Kouzes & Posner, 2011). Rather than getting lost in the past or future, we can choose to more intentionally focus on the present moment by listening deeply, fostering an environment that inspires greater trust and authenticity, with less judgment and negativity toward others (Berns-Zare, 2023b). This respectful communication process acknowledges the uniqueness and value of others and reduces habitual liking and not liking, approving and disapproving, and negative emotional reactions.

One communication strategy that can have a positive impact on relationships and teams is thoughtfully increasing the ratio of your positive statements compared to negative statements (Cameron, 2012; Losada & Heaphy, 2004). According to experts, sharing comments with a ratio of 3-6 positive statements for each one negative statement is an aspirational guideline that can strengthen relationships.

Many positive leaders use supportive communication strategies (Cameron, 2012). These tactics include sharing appreciation and encouragement when things are going well and endeavoring to preserve and support positive relationships when dealing with challenging or uncomfortable situations. Listening with greater mindfulness and compassion can empower each of us as leaders in our own lives and organizations, inspiring and supporting others, while also strengthening ourselves as positive role models and leaders.

Inspirations

Here are a few strategies to encourage supportive, mindful communication:

1 – **Speak and listen mindfully.**

- Be fully present to the conversation. Focus on the person who is speaking and listen actively.
- Pay attention to the speaker's reactions, in addition to the words. What do you see? What do you hear? What do you feel?
- Ask questions, listen to the speaker's response, and clarify your understanding as needed. For example: *"I heard you say…. Did I understand what you were saying?"*

- When you notice you're distracted, deliberately or mindfully pause, take a breath, and remind yourself to be fully present.

2 – Let yourself be flexible and open to ideas.

- Pause to notice and appreciate the efforts and strengths of others.
- Listen carefully to others' ideas and consider their viewpoints as you set goals and make decisions.
- When experiencing uncertainty, trust your strengths, experiences, and intuition as guideposts.
- Be patient and compassionate with yourself and others.
- Be open to considering new ideas and brainstorming "outside the box" beyond your typical lines of thinking.

3 – Act in your own best interest, while *also* respecting the rights of others.

- Listen carefully and respectfully with the intention to understand others.
- Speak clearly and firmly with a steady, calm voice.
- Be aware of your body language. Make eye contact in a way that feels comfortable and with the intention to be respectful of others and with awareness of cultural differences.

4 – Offer more positive than negative messages in conversations.

- Initiate feedback with the intention of strengthening and building relationships.
- Where it's appropriate, you might choose to show encouragement and appreciation. For example: *"Can you say more?" "This is a good idea," "You make a valid point here," "I appreciate your hard work on this."*
- When you offer negative messages, be supportive, maintaining respect for the other person. Try to be clear and concise, considering the other person's feelings as well as your own. For example, *"I can see you've worked hard on this. Now what can you do to solve the one remaining challenge?"*

This week I will experiment with one strategy to communicate more mindfully.

CHAPTER 43

Folding Positive
Emotions into Your Day

One sunny spring day, I was painting a gate and small fence in our yard. Paint brushes, paint cans, and large sheets of the local newspaper covered the ground around me. While I was immersed in the fourth hour of a task that I'd mistakenly thought would take about an hour, my friend called. In that same moment, a robust, unexpected wind gust blew itself into the calm, windless morning, slamming my wet, half-painted gate shut and scattering loose newspapers everywhere.

My immediate go-to reaction in this situation might typically be exasperation, but that's not how this scene played out. "Oh, my goodness!" I exclaimed to my friend on the phone as I narrated what was happening. Then, I laughed aloud at the chaos, and so did she. Deep inside me, I knew that laughing at that situation would have been her go-to response, and instinctively I mirrored a similar reaction. A moment later, I began gathering up the mess and continued painting, all the while chatting with her on the phone.

Rather than negativity, this potentially annoying experience awakened positive emotions – joy, amusement, and perhaps serenity contextualized within a social bond of love. A challenging moment during a mundane task offered a surprising invitation to turn toward positivity and thrive in the process.

Yes, negativity and unpleasant emotions often come spontaneously and are easy to generate. For example: anger, frustration, hostility, hurt, bitterness, finding fault. However, in many circumstances, the potential for positivity is also available (Berns-Zare, 2023c). For me, this experience turned out to be a great opportunity to transform frustration and anger to amusement and a positive moment.

Choosing positive emotions can not only help us rebound from setbacks. They can also help us connect with others more readily and discover alternate possibilities for creating a healthier, more vibrant life (Fredrickson, 2009; Roth & Laireiter, 2021). This concept is *not* about ignoring negative emotions or pretending they don't exist. Of course, we experience difficulties, obstacles, and losses, and it can be important to acknowledge them and the emotions that accompany the experiences. But in many situations, the potential for choosing a pleasant emotion, at least in the moment, is also available. Consider the possibility you have options about how you choose to respond. Will you choose a pleasant emotion or an unpleasant emotion in a particular moment?

Based on her team's extensive research over more than two decades, Barbara Fredrickson (2009) summarized a top 10 list of positive emotions that occur most frequently: (1) joy, (2) gratitude, (3) serenity, (4) interest, (5) hope, (6) pride, (7) amusement, (8) inspiration, (9) awe, and (10) love.

Inspirations

What if you could fold one or more additional moments of positive emotions into your days? These positive emotions are common in human experience, and they are available to everyone. A lot depends on how you think about an experience or situation. By intentionally choosing to notice a particular experience through an alternate lens with a more positive mindset, you can add more positive emotions to your life.

Here's an experiment you might want to try:

For just one or two minutes each day this week, aim to experience a positive emotion in a situation where you might not have noticed the opportunity before. When something happens during the day that you typically would not pay attention to, or might experience negatively, try noticing it through a more positive lens, folding in a moment or two that includes one of the ten positive emotions (joy, gratitude, serenity, interest, hope, pride, amusement, inspiration, awe, love) or another positive emotion. Then, simply invite yourself to pause and notice your experience.

For example:

You're walking hurriedly outdoors when you notice a small patch of flowers growing. Do you walk by or stop and notice? Potential positive emotions: awe, interest, serenity.

A struggling parent with a whining child is near you in the check-out line at the grocery store. You smile and the child smiles back. Potential positive emotions: amusement, joy, love.

The car in front of you stops abruptly and you're able to brake in time to avoid a collision. Potential positive emotions: gratitude, joy.

***This week I will practice folding one
additional positive emotion into my days,
where I might not have noticed one before.***

CHAPTER 44

Lighting Your Path As
You Dance with Change

The paths we walk in our lives from young adulthood to midlife to older adulthood are filled with varying blends of wholeness and vulnerability, clarity and confusion, resilience and resignation, meaning and meaninglessness, light and darkness.

At each stage of personal development from childhood to old age, we encounter gifts and challenges. Many of life's experiences are common to all of us. Other experiences may be more unique as we bring our personal selves to the lives we live. Each stage offers choice points, opportunities to discern and invigorate our purpose as we aspire toward the person we want to be.

In contemplating the second half of life, terms like *life reinvention, aging well, vibrancy, aging wisely, elderhood,* and *prime time* can offer guideposts for navigating transitions, changes, and development. These terms frame midlife and beyond with an eye toward opportunities, continued learning, and processes that can evoke resilience, awareness, and growth, rather than simply declines and endings. While we cannot escape life's suffering and losses, we *can* sharpen our skills for seeking experiences of happiness, meaning, and wisdom regardless of our circumstances.

It can be helpful to remember that everyone and everything changes. Transitions and changes occur inside each of us and all around us, in our relationships, workplaces, professions, communities, and throughout the natural world. Typically, we welcome some changes and rebel against others.

How do you meet life's transitions and changes? Do you dance with the changes or run away and try to hide?

One way to understand change is by considering the concept of three phases of change (Bridges, 2009):

Phase 1 is *the ending*. Letting go of the old situation. Acknowledging and dealing with the endings, losses, or shifts. Phase 2 is *the transition or in-between* time, the wilderness between the old reality of what was and the new beginning. This may be a time of many feelings, such as disorientation, sadness, confusion, distress, joy, or relief. And Phase 3 is the *new beginning*, figuring out how to make the change work and finding tactics to embrace the new way.

As you navigate your life, although you may have little or no control over outside events, you can choose where you direct your attention and the attitudes you bring to your experiences. You can make choices that either bolster or undermine the flow of your experience as you face endings, transitions, and new beginnings.

Inspirations

If you are experiencing a transition or change, whether invited or unwelcome, let yourself recognize it. Feel what you need to feel. Consider sharing your experiences and related emotions, thoughts, and reactions with people you trust.

To some degree, how you experience your life depends on your perspective. Do you see the many transitions and changes of midlife and beyond as a time for continued development or a time of decline? Do you embrace self-discovery, reinvention, resilience, and new beginnings amid life's shifts and challenges?

Here are some inspirations to light your path as you dance with change in this season of your life:

- Pay attention to your physical health and well-being. Get enough rest, take a walk outdoors, enjoy nature.
- Remember your sense of humor. Laughter and noticing the lighter side of a situation can be effective allies to help you soothe tension and stress.
- Experience learning something new or trying something new every day.
- Pause for moments of prayer, contemplation, contemplative movement, or mindfulness.
- Wake up early and watch the sunrise or settle down to watch the sunset.
- Let go of an old negative thought that no longer serves the quality of your life, and if an item no longer serves you, can you share, donate, sell, or discard it?
- Engage in acts of kindness, compassion, or social activism. Even small actions have the potential to make a positive difference.
- Remember you have this moment right now. Invite yourself to pause and notice it.
- When you are ready, consider your next steps. Set SMART goals: *Specific and clear, Measurable, Attainable, Relevant and Time-bound.* Then take one or more manageable steps to move forward.

This week I will honor my experience of change and choose an inspirational practice to light my path in this season of my life.

CHAPTER 45

Continuing to Learn

As I write this chapter, I remember my father who passed away a few years ago. My dad was a good man who lived a long, productive life. He was not so much a man of words as a man of action, a man of doing, who helped me learn.

My dad taught me how to play catch and hit a baseball. He helped me learn how to ride a two-wheeler by running along beside me and letting go at the right time. Dad was honest, hard-working, and there for us when we needed him.

Dad could fix almost anything, and if he didn't know how, he would learn. He built a bike for me when I was about nine years old. He found a frame, painted it the color I requested, fire engine red, and assembled it with new fenders. And he put on a new silver banana seat and high handlebars with red and white streamers hanging from each end. Other kids got new 3-speed racers, and I got the bike my dad built. I was never completely sure what to make of that, but I always knew my dad crafted it with love, and it was fun to help him.

A few years before the ravages of dementia stole the best parts of his mind, Dad told me about an article he'd read in *Readers Digest* magazine when I was growing up. He explained that he didn't know much about how to be a good father, so he'd read articles in newspapers, and this magazine to help him learn to become a better parent to my brother and me.

I miss my dad. As I reflect on his life and that conversation, I understand with greater clarity the many ways to learn in our lives. Earlier in this book, I offered some ideas about the concept of a growth mindset. People with a growth mindset believe we can change and perform better through our learning and experience (Dweck, 2006). Through our efforts and belief in our capacity to grow, we can rise to life's challenges more effectively.

Like my dad, we all have opportunities to learn and develop each day.

Inspirations

These strategies are stirred by my dad's wisdom. Is there one or more you'd like to experiment with this?

1-Listen actively in conversations. We can learn a lot from kids, colleagues, peers, and the person who sits next to us on the bus or airplane. We often learn more by listening than speaking.

2-Ask for honest feedback and get good at receiving it.

3-Take advantage of opportunities to read, attend workshops, listen to webinars, or take a class. When you learn something that you want to remember, create a prompt or note to remind you. Carry these takeaways into your life.

4-Listen to the messages from your heart, your gut, and your inner voice. Some of the answers lie in the heart of your being. Deep inside yourself, you know what you need and what really matters.

5-Get into action toward something you want to achieve. Set goals for yourself, and use to-do lists to stay focused.

6-Seek nuggets of wisdom from your observations and experiences. How can you turn a setback into an opportunity? Remember there are often opportunities to learn from others and also from what we see, hear, feel, and know deep within ourselves.

7-Try new things. For example, try a game, recipe, or a new skill, plant a vegetable garden, care for the earth, sing, dance, learn a new language, or start a conversation with an acquaintance.

Do you believe that your efforts and experiences can lead to change, transformation, and building your abilities over time?   How can you challenge yourself to grow in your life?

This week I will consider my beliefs about learning and challenge myself to learn something new.

CHAPTER 46

Awakening What Matters to You

What are the central questions in your life? What meaningful questions are you contemplating, or do you want to contemplate?

The *big* questions we reflect on can inspire and empower our life's journey. As we strengthen our steps at midlife and beyond, our contemplative self-inquiries can gently nudge or strongly awaken mind, body, and spirit. Although we may not have the answers, these questions can bring meaning and shape to our lives. For some of us, questions unfold and shift through our experiences as time moves forward, while for others, the questions hold steady while the answers slowly evolve.

Meaning, purpose, and mattering are influential building blocks for happiness and thriving personally and at work (Kellerman & Seligman 2023; Seligman, 2011). According to mounting evidence, exploring purpose in life promotes well-being and healthy aging. A study of over 6000 people revealed that having a sense of purpose may even help us live longer (Hill & Turiano, 2014). Participants in the study responded to several statements as a barometer of well-being, including "Some people wander aimlessly through life, but I am not one of them." Findings indicated that people who reported a higher sense of purpose experienced greater longevity. Data also pointed to the importance of a strong sense of purpose at younger ages. It's important to note that exploring meaningful directions in earlier life can contribute to a positive quality of life as we get older.

Uncovering what really matters typically involves stepping back from day-to-day and considering life through a broader, deeper perspective. There's no single meaning, goal, or ideal that fits for everyone. The source of purpose and meaning varies greatly among individuals and it can change across the lifespan. Within the complexities of our lives, what we experience as meaningful and fulfilling may shift and transform as we do.

Inspirations

What central questions call to you as you consider what matters in your life? I invite you to choose one or more of these self-inquires or any others to reflect on for inspiration (Berns-Zare, 2017). In this process you might want to pause, step back, and adjust your longer lens. Chapter 27 may offer a useful companion for reflection and discernment. You might find it helpful to speak the questions and your responses aloud, or write them in your notebook, journal, or electronic device.

Ideas for Questions to Awaken Your Sense of Meaning

- What really matters to me?
- To be myself, what do I need to do or to be?
- If I were writing a book about my life's story, what would the title be? What do I *wish* the title of my autobiography could be?
- When I listen to the quiet voice inside me, what do I hear, see, and feel?
- If I could change three things about my life, what would they be?
- If I were five times more courageous, what would I do?
- Is there another question that you want to ask and respond to?

Questions to Call Yourself to Action

- What small actions can I take to become more of the person I want to be?
- What goal would I like to set for myself and work on to completion?
- Which of my priorities may change, if I choose to pursue this objective?

- What would it require of me if I chose to create action toward this goal?
- What action steps am I ready to take today? This week? This month?

This week I will consider one or more big questions to awaken what matters to me.
When I am ready, I will call myself to action.

CHAPTER 47

The Courage to Accept
that We Are Enough

I am not perfect, and I know it. I've been aware of my vulnerability, imperfections, and flawed humanity as far back as I can remember. Here's today's difference. I used to think of my imperfectness as something that would go away when I "grew up." The saddest and most uncomfortable aspect was the fear that I was more imperfect, more broken, than most people, which sometimes made me feel different and an outsider.

During my graduate school studies, I explored the classic book *On Becoming a Person*, by renowned humanistic psychologist Carl Rogers (1961). Dr. Rogers' lifetime of research and experiential work highlighted compassion and self-empowerment as rich resources to help us stretch toward our fullest potential. He shared his own experience with imperfection, offering the concept of enough-ness and the empowerment of knowing that being human *is* enough. Many times, throughout the years, I've returned to these teachings. If Carl Rogers could accept that he was imperfect, why couldn't I?

I also studied the writings of Viktor Frankl about finding meaning in even the most difficult circumstances. As a Holocaust survivor, Dr. Frankl deeply understood the freedom to choose our attitude in any situation, and that this choice can help us discover meaning in our lives (Frankl, 1985). He wrote that our responses, rather than the conditions in which we find ourselves, determine who we are. Dr. Frankl's writings have been critical for my own contemplative reflections and have enlightened my evolving relationship with personal vulnerability.

More recently, via the contemporary research of Brené Brown I am discovering resources for further inspiration and courage. Dr. Brown describes imperfection as a gift (Brown, 2010). In her book, *The Gifts of Imperfection*, she writes about authenticity and letting ourselves know we are enough. She explains that we are all imperfect—not just you and me, but all of us—and she explores the gifts of our brokenness, including compassion, connection, and courage. As we reflect, seeking to understand and discern these big ideas, we can choose to let go of who we "should" be and engage who we truly are.

Inspirations

Learning to courageously accept your wholeness and enough-ness, along with noticing the beauty in your vulnerability, brokenness, and imperfections can offer you daily opportunities to welcome your true self. Here are a few inspirational ideas. Perhaps there is one or more that you may want to ponder as you explore your enough-ness:

- I have choices about how I see myself, and I do *not* have to suffer with negative self-talk. While I may not be perfect, I am enough, worthy of love, belonging, and connection.
- I am resilient and have internal and external resources to draw from.
- My breath is my aliveness. With each breath, I am enough. Wherever I am, I can simply notice one breath at a time. There is no need to change how I am breathing. I observe each breath with calmness and clarity. I am worthy. I am present. I am enough.
- I am not alone in the hidden wholeness of this interconnected world.

This week I will remember that I have choices about how I see myself and remind myself that while I am not perfect, I am enough.

CHAPTER 48

Recognizing the Infinite
Worth of Ourselves and Others

During life's difficult times, it can feel like our world is floundering and we are too small to make a difference. At the same time, in the second half of life many of us grow more conscious of the wisdom of our experience and maturity, along with an enlivened awareness of the value of every life.

The 21st century is offering new opportunities to explore the intersection of science, psychology, spirituality, and personal exploration. Revolutionary scientific findings in quantum physics show that our essential reality is *not* material (Miskovic & Lynn, 2025; Ponte & Schafer, 2013; Swimme & Berry, 1992). There is much we cannot see, invisible realities that exist, and new understandings about the mysteries that connect everyone and everything. These new understandings from empirical science and contemplative wisdom can shift how we experience ourselves and the world around us.

Contemplating the idea that our lives are somehow interwoven, that all of us matter, that everyone is born with infinite worth, can remind us of the interconnections of all humanity. The 13th century Sufi philosopher, Jalal al-Din Rumi, suggested that we give birth to ourselves slowly (Rumi & Barks, 1995). These awakenings can offer pathways to ponder a broader experience about who we are, creating new connections and dialogues as we pay attention to our inner wisdom, invigorating the wholeness that unites the common ground of our humanity.

Sociologist Parker Palmer recommends that we slow down, sit quietly, and learn how to be present with others in ways that can help us regain our sense of who we truly are and evoke community (2024). And I wonder about ways to open to the profound understanding that every one of us is inherently worthy of love and to the hope that repairing our broken world is possible.

Our essential true selves and the true wholeness of others invite us to truly honor each other with kindness and compassion (Margolius, 2018). What would life be like if more of us could begin to generate human acts of kindness, from the smallest daily interactions to the larger acts of social justice? Two of the many pathways for honoring life's infinite worth are practicing mindfulness and becoming aware of our strengths. Practicing mindfulness builds our capacity for awareness of our present moment with less negativity and judgment. Being aware of our character strengths and using them in positive ways can invigorate our well-being and support our efforts to contribute to repairing a world that values human life.

In Chapter 12, you learned about the 24 character strengths identified by positive psychologists as gateways toward recognizing what's right with people (Niemiec, 2018; Peterson & Seligman, 2004). Hope and kindness are two character strengths that can energize our awareness. Hope, or future-mindedness, involves visualizing a good future and working to achieve it. Kindness is care, generosity, and compassion for others.

Inspirations

If you'd like to energize your awareness of the infinite worth of yourself and others, here are a few inspirational ideas:

1- Sit in silence for a mindful moment or more. Pause and notice the flow of your breath (in-breath, out-breath), or choose another anchor. Ask yourself how you can generate even a moment of kindness or hope toward yourself or another person today. Repeat this mindful moment each day (or several days) this week.

2- Identify a focus phrase to support your valuing of human life (Margolius, 2018). Post this phrase in a visible location where you'll see it frequently. Here are a few examples: *"I am enough and can make a positive difference." "You are filled with infinite light, as am I." "I am worthy and part of our interconnected world."*

3-Over three or four days this week, contemplate one or more of these questions or others that you find meaningful in this book. You might choose to use your journal, notebook, or electronic device to help you open your thoughts more expressively and write them down (Pennebaker & Smyth, 2016).

- When have I noticed or experienced the hope or kindness of others? What was this experience like for me? How did I feel and what did I learn about myself, others, or the world?
- How do I feel when I am engaging in hope or kindness?
- How can I experience more hope or be more kind toward myself?
- How can I express hope or kindness in interactions with others?

4-Engage in meaningful conversations to explore some of these ideas and seek areas of common ground. Create a space of safety to share ideas. Talk with other people about what the infinite worth of each person means to them and to you. Discuss strategies to bring kindness into the spaces you share: families, friendships, community groups, and the people at work. Ask questions, explore ideas, listen carefully and deeply. For more on leading with supportive, mindful conversations, see Chapter 42 of this book.

Wherever you are in the lifespan, there are opportunities to recognize the infinite worth of others and yourself and life's interconnections. Even in the simplest ways, you can bring greater kindness and hope to the world.

This week I will ponder my awareness of who I truly am, and experiment with an inspirational strategy to light my way.

CHAPTER 49

Living Beyond the Everyday

In the second half of life, many of us begin to drink from a deeper well, becoming aware that there is more to life than what we can see with our eyes. The adventures that arise from this *something more* evolve from our personal journeys and carry different meanings for each of us.

We might assume we'll grow more aware and wiser, more courageous and compassionate simply as a product of our accumulated years, but it's not that simple for most of us. The process of awakening our understandings of who we are and who we can become is a pilgrimage that begins at birth and continues throughout the meandering paths of our lives.

Since my youth, I've wondered about the world beyond what my eyes could see. As a teen, I recall telling a friend while we walked along the Lake Michigan shoreline that I saw my life as "the search." I wondered about questions like, "Why am I here?" "What is my purpose in life?" and "Why do things happen as they do?" Fast forward to my late 50's when the inquiry "What shall I do with this precious life?" propelled my thoughts, studies, career, and practices on a path that I'd scarcely imagined. These flowing inquiries continue to ebb and flow with vulnerabilities, awakenings, and as much courage as I can muster, as I explore transformative possibilities and new pathways that fit my ways of being in the world.

What I would call a guiding inspiration on my journey is the idea that many answers to life's big questions lie at the heart of our beings, that deep inside ourselves we come to know what really matters to us as individuals and in life's bigger picture. In my experience, I would characterize the process of these wanderings as an ever-expanding expedition and an ongoing process of learning to discern between doing and being. I aspire toward living in the light with vitality. I yearn to remember to pause and *mindfully* notice and appreciate more moments as they occur, rather than wandering *mindlessly* in the sometimes overwhelming busyness of everyday life.

Today's 21st century is unprecedented in our world. Our intentions, choices, and actions matter greatly as we navigate roles as leaders and elders in our families, friendships, and communities. Yet at varying vantage points amid our passages through life, we may observe that we're part of something much larger in the universal grand scheme, and these observations can carry different meanings for different people.

There are many ways we can come to know and learn. There are the objective teachings of science and logic and also the realms of personal observations, experience, intuitions, and consciousness. While science and logic have been studied more intensively, the more personal realms have had little exploration by researchers (Miskovic & Lynn, 2025). Rather, these experiences are more speculative and phenomenological, that is, based on our own experiences and personal ways of being in the world. It is for each of us to explore and glean understandings about where our personal experiences and understandings fit within the frameworks through which we see ourselves, each other, and the world.

For many of us, spiritual explorations are among the great quests of our lives. Experts across disciplines have observed that spirituality, broadly defined as searching to discover the sacred and transcendent, is a universal phenomenon, crossing cultures throughout the world. Many of us occasionally glimpse a mysterious sense of something greater than we are that seems to unite us in some benevolent way. Although the content may vary, spirituality typically involves a compassionate, transcendent experience of connecting with humanity and the natural world (Dalai Lama & Cutler, 1998; Easvaradoss & Rajan, 2013; Peterson, 2006; Peterson & Seligman, 2004).

In most cultures throughout history, spirituality has been an aspect of human life. Research studies have linked spirituality to happiness, positive social relationships, life satisfaction, sense of purpose and meaning, self-regulation, and the capacity to cope with stress and illness (Easvaradoss & Rajan, 2013; Niemiec, 2018; Zagano & Gillespie, 2006). And there are many related opportunities to express spirituality through other strengths including gratitude, forgiveness, kindness, love, and appreciation of beauty and excellence.

On your own journey through life, have you ever noticed glimmers of understanding and wisdom that feel transformative or significant in some larger way?

The trek through midlife and beyond offers varied moments for growing inspiration and experiencing personal inner unfoldment. There are many ways this can happen. We may catch glimpses of the essence of our being or experience moments of awe in nature. We may explore meaning and purpose in our lives. We may connect meaningfully with others. We may ponder the deeper wisdom of our experiences. We may expand our understandings as we learn from the world's spiritual traditions, contemplative reflections, scientific explorations, inspirational teachers, and our own personal practices.

In addition, life offers many opportunities to cultivate our own unfolding as we reach out in connection and service to others via relationships and community. The term *spiritual eldering* describes a process that not only can offer well-being, meaning, and purpose to elders but also share our wisdom and ideas with future generations (Schechter-Shalomi & Miller, 1995). The seasons of our lives can flow with greater meaning, well-being, and new understandings as we notice life in new ways, explore beyond the everyday, ask life's big questions, and contemplate our roles in the transpersonal wholeness of all.

Reflecting on life's *big* questions can be transformative. Exploring big questions can awaken your intuitive capacities, light up your internal compass, and catalyze your ways of being present in your daily life. They can offer a springboard toward taking action to create a better world.

And deep personal questions can help you learn to pause instead of just reacting, listen to your inner knowing, and perhaps make wiser choices.

Inspirations

This week you are invited to reflect on the idea that there may be more to life beyond the everyday. Here are a few questions to inspire your exploration.

- Where do you find inspiration? Do you feel inspired by nature, practicing mindfulness, seeking meaning in the present moment, moments of awe, reading spiritual or inspirational books, engaging in reflection or prayer, connecting meaningfully with others, feeling fully immersed in the flow of a task or activity, contributing to a cause you believe in, or other ways?
- How are your ideas and choices guided by a sense of something larger than yourself?
- Where does spirituality fit in your life currently? How, if at all, would you like to transform the role of spirituality in your life?
- What's one way you are or could be a spiritual elder? A few examples include volunteering, working for a cause you believe in, mentoring or simply listening empathically to a child, adolescent, or young adult, or showing compassion to another person.
- How can you create time to engage in reflection or inspirational practice this week?

This week I will unfold my spiritual map and open to possibilities larger than myself.

CHAPTER 50

Engagement, Flow, and
Resilience in Your Daily Life

Each of my grandchildren has played baseball or softball in their young lives. We enjoy watching them learn the game, play with their teammates, and develop their skills physically and emotionally. Yes, the game can be filled with fun and joy. And yet, this sport is not without its frustrations and challenges.

The game is fundamentally ingrained with bouts of adversity (Krause, 2023). A player stands in the batter's box ready to hit the ball but instead takes strikes or hits fouls. Then, there are times when a ball flies to the outfield and all eyes are on the lone fielder who misses or drops it. This game is inherent with pressures and failures, and my beloved offspring can attest to that. Yet, sport can also build resilience, engagement and *flow*, the sense of feeling fully immersed in an activity.

In these ways this game reflects daily life. Like it or not, our lives are filled with opportunities to strengthen our resilience and flow. Who, among us, doesn't encounter demands that strain our attention, abilities, and emotions? Life pitches lots of strikes, testing our ability to respond to pressures, setbacks, and difficulties. As we struggle to get back up when we fall, we discover that confronting adversity is an expectable part of human experience, whether playing in a ball game or in the day-to-day of our lives.

Resilience is a key theme in this book. Why? Because at any age, the ability to respond and adapt in the face of adversity can be a protective buffer, helping us persevere and adapt amid tough times. Resilience can help us bounce back when we strike out, miss the mark, or fall down in the game of life. It doesn't chase away our problems, but it can help us see beyond them and handle them more effectively.

Yet, there's more to life than simply adapting to adversity. While we need to respond to life's challenges, we can also benefit from appreciating our experiences as they occur and aspire to see the panorama beyond them. Our experiences can be much more fulfilling when we are doing something that holds our attention in some positive way, inviting us to focus and fully engage, creating greater efficacy, satisfaction, and a more rewarding experience. Engagement or flow is a key component of wellbeing, flourishing, and happiness in life (Seligman, 2011).

So, let's turn to the game of life, more specifically the second half of life. In our busy lives, we often become distracted and may not pay attention to what we're doing. Even when we are doing good stuff, we may not truly enjoy it because we're feeling stressed or worried about something that has already happened or might occur in the future. We aren't fully present to what is happening and miss noticing positive experiences here and now because we're distracted or focused elsewhere.

One way to create a more optimal experience, to feel a deeper sense of enjoyment is to invest our attention in a way that increases the experience of engagement or flow (Csikszentmihalyi, 1990). It's even possible to experience flow even during difficulties. Dr. Csikszentmihalyi says a key trait of people who can experience engagement during adversity is "non-self-conscious individualism," described as internal motivation not easily distracted by outside circumstances or events. With flow, we can learn to compensate for weaknesses. Paying careful attention to relevant details, we can find hidden opportunities to set goals, take action, monitor progress and learn from it, and then gradually set bigger goals and challenges for ourselves.

I have a friend who recently had knee surgery. She gets up to walk several times each day. The first day she walked about five steps, the next day ten steps, paying focused attention to her balance, movement, and even her breath. Now, she is up to walking almost a quarter of a mile outdoors and enjoying the beauty of the summer gardens and sunshine. She told me that once she got so absorbed by the emerging rhythms of her careful steps, she lost track of time and walked a bit longer than she had planned. It's not glamourous, but she is engaged amid adversity, engaged in the flow of her experience.

Inspirations

Can you think of an activity you find so absorbing, pleasurable or meaningful that when you are engaging in it time seems to stand still?

Experiencing a sense of flow in activities you like involves a strong focus on what you are doing, a sense of being immersed or being in the zone. To move toward flow, you can invite yourself to pay attention to what's happening now, responding to setbacks and continuing to progress toward your objective. There is a sense that your skills can meet the challenge of the activity or at least that the objective is potentially in your range of control (Hays, 2024; Johnson, 2021).

There are many ways to experience flow. This kind of engagement involves focusing keenly on what you're doing. This can happen when you are doing routine activities, working, playing, or doing something fun, creative, meaningful, or something else. Flow can happen when you are performing, playing an instrument, walking, meditating, praying, washing the dishes, exercising, or even rehabbing from an injury.

According to experts, it doesn't matter what the goal is, flow is typically goal-directed so it's important to have an objective and want to achieve it (Csikszentmihalyi, 1990; Hays, 2004). Choosing a goal that is meaningful, compelling in some way, and within your range of ability can bolster your experience of flow and optimal experience. And it's helpful to discern a good balance between your goal and your perception of your level of ability to address the challenges you are engaged in.

With intentionality, *you* can learn to bring greater flow into your life. Flow is facilitated by engaging in enjoyable tasks that your body can do. Whether softball, baseball, pickleball or another sport, singing, dancing, hiking, walking, writing, arts and crafts, or something else, find an activity that can offer you moments of engagement or pleasure. Other examples include reading a good book, engaging in a compelling hobby, playing a game you enjoy, gardening, practicing your golf swing, swimming, woodworking, doing yoga or needlework.

Recently, I took a basketweaving class, something I had never done before. The instructor assured us we would all finish the day with a beautiful basket that we wove ourselves. I felt that the required skills were within my ability to learn, and I loved the creativity and social connection in the group. Thus, I became so absorbed that I felt completely engaged in the task, and my goal of completing the basket. I was the last one to finish making my basket, but I completed it. Looking back at the end of day, I realized that this had been a flow experience.

This week I will intentionally endeavor to experience a sense of flow in an activity, paying attention to my engagement in a way that brings me enjoyment.

CHAPTER 51

Exploring Your Big Questions
in an Interconnected World

We live in an interconnected world much larger than ourselves as individuals. We are born into communities of all kinds. Throughout our lives, we perpetually bump up against life's many circumstances, influencing and interrupting us in a myriad of ways, even when we are unaware of their impact. Sometimes, we are confronted with impacts that are unescapable, mingling good with bad, connection with disconnection, and gains with losses.

Throughout the interrelated conditions of our existences, we try to live our story as best we can. We stumble around among what we come into the world with and the surroundings in which we find ourselves. Intentionally or unintentionally, we try to find some kind of balance across relationships, events, and the passage of time that fits with how we see ourselves. Put more academically, as humans, we are shaped by our own internal individual factors (what goes on inside us) and by social systems, the broader external and contextual factors that surround us near and far. For example, family, neighborhood, workplace, communities, country, and the earth.

We humans are social beings, and the many *contexts of our lives* are complex, impacting on our wellbeing, resilience, ideas, behaviors, and much more. Although we're essentially here as individuals on our own, our growth and development are influenced by the layers of systems that surround us. These environmental circumstances shape our personal and communal relationships, cultural beliefs, social norms, politics, customs, traditions, and laws.

Our inner experiences and actions are inspired by our interactions with the many and varied levels of the interconnected human environmental systems in which we live (Bronfenbrenner, 1994). As individuals, these interconnections can be visualized as concentric rings with you at the center. Then, additional layers expand outward toward the progressively broader world. The layers include your immediate contexts, such as intimate relationships, family, neighborhood, workplace, and wider structures of society, such as cultures, religions/spiritual traditions, communities, and countries. More than you may realize, your internal (personal) ideas, values, and development are deeply intertwined with these layers of externals.

In these turbulent times, our world is shifting in many ways. Yet, at the same time, the world is abundant, filled with beauty and light. Recognizing these contexts can help you understand how events around you may influence your own feelings, reactions, and internal dialogues. Wellbeing practices, such as those we've explored in this book, can help you navigate your journey as you engage with the world around you. As you seek to further develop the skills to flourish in your life, you can also remember to pay careful attention to the natural world. You can notice nature's profound harmonies and dynamics, appreciating why they matter. Whether you are planting flowers in your window, observing nature and natural surroundings with awe, or caring for the earth, you can gain greater awareness of the natural world that is vital for your very survival.

Whether you are engaging in relationships, or noticing moments with mindfulness and gratitude, these and many other habits and practices can offer you greater resilience and wellbeing as you recognize the innumerable ways humanity is intertwined with the planet on which we live.

Of course, our personal journeys are mingled with joy and challenges in each season of our lives. While we may have little or no control over many of the external contexts in which we live, we do have some measure of influence over how we choose to engage with the circumstances and events that ripple through our lives. We are the authors of our stories and the legacies we leave to future generations.

Inspirations

The poet Mary Oliver (2017) famously asks us in her poem, "The Summer Day," to intentionally consider how we want to engage with our untamed and precious existence. The questions you ask yourself, and how you respond to them, can influence who you are and who you might become. Your story is yours to live out and to share in the context of your own life and all the contexts in which you find yourself. What is your life inviting you to—to be present to, to speak, to share the gifts that are yours in this interconnected world?

Here are a few self-inquiry questions to help you find your way:

- What makes your life precious to you and to others?
- What big questions do you ask yourself?
- What are some of the layers and components of your environment? For example: family, friends, organizations, schools, local government, work, income sources?
- What do you notice about the ways you're affected by the layers of your environment?
- What do you value and how true are you to what you value in the ways you live your life?
- What thoughts and emotions are awakened as you ponder your responses to these questions?
- What would you want to learn more about?
- What do you think you *should* learn more about?
- What haven't you done *yet* that you really want to engage in?
- If you were to do this, how would it fit with what you value and your sense of purpose?
- In what way might you want to find a new pathway going forward?
- What are you waiting for?

As you approach the end of this book, you are invited to look back at some of the questions you have explored. Which questions from this chapter and others in the book stand out to you as you live the story of your life and perhaps reimagine new possibilities? What questions do you want to continue to reflect on as you go forward?

This week I will continue to reflect on questions that matter to me and consider which ones I want to take forward with me into the story of my life.

CHAPTER 52

Reimagining Midlife and Beyond: Practices to Invigorate Your Resilience and Wellbeing

This book's final chapter offers a summary of some of the strategies we've explored together. Whether you are reading this book in its entirety or skimming the chapters that catch your attention, I hope you are finding some ideas that you resonate with and choose to carry into your precious life to energize greater wholeness and wellbeing.

As we navigate midlife and beyond, there are many opportunities to discover the expansiveness of our individual potential, reach toward greater fulfillment, and contribute to the world around us from the best of ourselves.

The act of living is a process, *not* a destination. As we experience life, we explore our unique ways of being in the world in the changing seasons of our lives (Kaufman, 2020; Rogers, 1995). The situations and our responses will vary. Each of us needs to find our own way as we discover what strategies inspire and resonate with us. Whatever our fundamental capacities, strengths, and experiences, living with greater resilience and well-being is possible for each of us. Every emerging day offers 1,440 new moments of possibility to invigorate our potential and our presence in this vast, mysterious, interconnected world.

Many philosophers, psychologists, and spiritual teachers offer ideas and formulas to inspire us to live a good life, a flourishing life, a meaningful life. I resonate greatly with the concept that in the big picture perhaps the best we can offer is to walk each other home with compassion and our presence (Dass & Bush, 2018). I see this idea as an aspirational calling and a poignant reminder that what matters greatly is to be ourselves, to show up, and live as best we can while trying in some way to bring goodness to the world. And a sense of humor doesn't hurt either.

As we journey through the middle and later seasons of our lives, we will each decide what a good life means for us. For many, living with meaning is an essential aspiration—*not* just living with pleasure for pleasure's sake but rather exploring practices that help you develop toward your whole self and full humanity (Kaufman, 2020; Maslow, 1987; Wong, 2016). The practices in this book offer a wellspring of inspiration to help you infuse your life in ways you find invigorating, meaningful, and transformative.

Here are some of the inspirational ideas and evidence-informed strategies explored in this book that may offer guideposts as you explore this season of your life and those to come. What choices will you make to empower yourself and bolster your well-being in the day-to-day of your life?

- **Live with more mindful presence.** Pause. Gently pay attention to the moments of your life.
- **Create a positivity list.** Identify five things that lift your spirits and, as you can, include them in your life.
- **Find ways to engage in flow.** Let yourself feel fully engaged in activities that you enjoy and are meaningful to you.
- **Be kind.** Show compassion to others, and be compassionate with yourself.
- **Reach out and connect with others.** Relationships, even brief interactions, can contribute to flourishing and overall wellbeing.
- **Leverage your strengths.** Your top strengths could be thought of as your superpowers. Engage them to energize yourself and power up your life.
- **Set meaningful goals.** Act mindfully on clear, realistic objectives.

- **Muster up your grit.** Practice effectively and steadfastly toward your goal, even when you feel like giving up.
- **Savor positive experiences.** Notice good moments, such as experiences of joy, comfort, or beauty. Celebrate good news.
- **Build your vitality.** Get as active as you are able, for example, walking, using the stairs, or gardening.
- **Remember to laugh.** Stretch your smile muscles each day. Find ways to add humor into your days.
- **Dance with transitions and changes.** Your choices can either bolster or undermine your experience as you face endings, turning points, and new beginnings.
- **Continue learning and growing.** Approach life with curiosity and a beginner's mindset. Try new things or do an everyday activity in a new way.
- **Practice gratitude.** Invite yourself to notice and be thankful for the goodness in your day-to-day life. Share gratitude with others.

What strategy is missing from this list that *you* would like to include?

Inspirations

Which of these strategies jumps out at you? Choose one practice you can commit to this week to create more well-being each day. Start with one clear, doable action. You might find it helpful to post the list as a reminder on your computer, refrigerator, or mirror. Or use the list to catch your attention as a bookmark in your favorite text or novel. What are your next steps?

This week I will empower my wellbeing as I experiment with one or more inspirational practices.

Concluding Thoughts:
Continuing the Journey

As we conclude our journey together through this book, let's revisit the idea we began with. You're *not* too old, and it's not too late to journey toward living as fully as you can in this season of your life.

Each of the 52 chapters in *You're Not Too Old and It's Not Too Late* offers an invitation to consider new possibilities at midlife and beyond. Perhaps you have found yourself reexamining your assumptions about growing older and considering new options as you envision your transitions, challenges, and opportunities now and in the years ahead.

Reawakening is a possibility in any moment. Living with greater meaning, mindfulness, and new possibilities is about figuring out how to engage in the best life you can in the face of life's joys and challenges. Considering how you can make choices to invigorate your mind, body, and spirit in the flow of your life. It's about awakening in the morning thinking about how to live today as fully as you are able. And ending the day, acknowledging the ups and the downs and exploring how you might choose to be present differently or what you might try to change tomorrow.

At the start of this book, I suggested forming a discussion group with a friend or a group of peers. One way to continue your journey and deepen your insights into the ideas and resources in this book would be to create a group framework, such as a flourishing circle or book group. This group, whether you meet in person or remotely, could help you explore the chapters with others, blending their responses with your own ideas, life experiences, and inspirations. Perhaps participants would choose to take turns facilitating the meetings. Chapter topics could be explored in any order for a week or over a period of several weeks, depending on your group's interests and choices.

I hope you have found this book an inspiring, invigorating companion on your path. I wish you inspiration, courage, and new possibilities as your journey continues.

Ilene Berns-Zare

www.ileneberns-zare.com

https://www.psychologytoday.com/us/contributors/ilene-berns-zare-psyd

https://www.linkedin.com/in/ilene-berns-zare-psyd-pcc-cec-9062a39b/

References

Achor, S. (2011, May). *The happy secret to better work* [Video]. TED Conferences. https://www.ted.com/talks/shawn_achor_the_happy_secret_to_better_work

Adler, L. P. (1998–2017). *National Centenarian Awareness Project.* https://www.adlercentenarians.com/

Alimujiang, A., Wiensch, A., Boss, J., Fleischer, N. L., Mondul, A. M., McLean, K., Mukherjee, B., & Pierce, C. L. (2019). Association between life purpose and mortality among US adults older than 50 years. *JAMA Network Open, 2*(5), e194270. https://jamanetwork.com/journals/jamanetworkopen/fullarticle/2734064

Amabile, T. M. (2019). Understanding retirement requires getting inside people's stories: A call for more qualitative research. *Work, Aging and Retirement, 5*(3), 207–211. https://doi.org/10.1093/workar/waz009

American Psychological Association. (2010, April). *Psychology of procrastination: Why people put off important tasks until the last minute.* https://www.apa.org/news/press/releases/2010/04/procrastination

American Psychological Association. (2014). *The road to resilience.* https://www.apa.org/helpcenter/road-resilience

American Psychological Association. (2024). *Stress in America 2024: A nation in political turmoil.* https://www.apa.org/pubs/reports/stress-in-america/2024

American Psychological Association. (2025). *Resilience.* https://www.apa.org/topics/resilience

Anderson-Lopez, K. A., & Lopez, R. (2019). *The next right thing* [Song recorded by Kristen Bell]. On *Frozen II* [Album]. Wonderland Music Company.

Arnett, J. J., Robinson, O., & Lachman, M. E. (2020). Rethinking adult development: Introduction to the special issue. *American Psychologist, 75*(4), 425–430. https://psycnet.apa.org/fulltext/2020-29966-001.html

Attia, P. (2023). *Outlive: The science and art of longevity.* Harmony.

Bandura, A. (1997). Self-efficacy: The exercise of control. W. H. Freeman & Co.

Baumeister, R. F. (1991). Meanings of life. Guilford Press.

Baumeister, R. F., Vohs, K. D., Asker, J. L., & Garbinsky, E. N. (2013). Some key differences between a happy life and a meaningful life. Journal of Positive Psychology, 8(6), 505–516. https://doi.org/10.1080/17439760.2013.830764.

Beaty, R. E. (2020). The creative brain. Cerebrum: The Dana Forum on Brain Science, 2020(cer-02-20). https://pubmed.ncbi.nlm.nih.gov/32206175/.

Berns-Zare, I. (2017). *25 powerful questions for awakening meaning in life and work: A guide to awareness and action.* https://ibzcoaching.com/25-powerful-questions-meaning-life-work/

Berns-Zare, I. (2018). *Just start: You don't have to like it to do it.* https://www.psychologytoday.com/us/blog/flourish-and-thrive/201811/just-start-you-dont-have-to-like-it-to-do-it

Berns-Zare, I. (2020a). *How to focus on what really matters: Using mindfulness moments to build resilience during COVID-19.* https://www.psychologytoday.com/us/blog/flourish-and-thrive/202004/how-focus-what-really-matters

Berns-Zare, I. (2020b). *Feeling anxious about a decision? Research reveals a powerful strategy for gaining greater clarity.* https://www.psychologytoday.com/us/blog/flourish-and-thrive/202007/feeling-anxious-about-a-decision

Berns-Zare, I. (2020c). 5 Keys to begin a positive shift in your life: Stop looking out there for answers. https://www.psychologytoday.com/us/blog/flourish-and-thrive/202011/5-keys-to-begin-a-positive-shift-in-your-life

Berns-Zare, I. (2020c). What keeps you up at night?: 5 tactics to tackle stress and reduce overwhelm. https://www.psychologytoday.com/us/blog/flourish-and-thrive/202001/what-keeps-you-night

Berns-Zare, I. (2020e). *6 powerful ways to build new habits: How strengthening your habits can strengthen your brain.* https://www.psychologytoday.com/us/blog/flourish-and-thrive/202002/6-powerful-ways-build-new-habit

Berns-Zare, I. (2023a). *Choosing less: An astounding way to have more – 4 questions to help you manage your wants and feel happier with what you have.* https://www.psychologytoday.com/us/blog/flourish-and-thrive/202309/choosing-less-an-astounding-way-to-have-more

Berns-Zare, I. (2023b). *Positive organisations: Mindful, compassionate leadership with a coaching mindset* [White paper]. Positive Psychology Guild. https://ppnetwork.org/positive-organisations-mindful-compassionate-leadership-with-a-coaching-mindset-by-ilene-berns-zare-psyd-white-paper/

Berns-Zare, I. (2023c). *Negativity or positivity? It's up to you.* https://www.psychologytoday.com/us/blog/flourish-and-thrive/202308/negativity-or-positivity-its-up-to-you

Berns-Zare, I. (2024). Creating meaningful personal rituals that inspire you. Powerful everyday actions can bring you greater awareness, connection, and joy. https://www.psychologytoday.com/us/blog/flourish-and-thrive/202412/creating-meaningful-personal-rituals-that-inspire-you

Berns-Zare, I. (2025). *The magic of learning from your experiences: How can you develop greater wisdom and resilience in day-to-day life?* https://www.psychologytoday.com/us/blog/flourish-and-thrive/202505/the-magic-of-learning-from-your-experiences

Biswas-Diener, R., & Dean, B. (2007). *Positive psychology coaching: Putting the science of happiness to work for your clients.* John Wiley & Sons.

Bonanno, G. A., & Keltner, D. (1997). Facial expressions of emotion and the course of conjugal bereavement. *Journal of Abnormal Psychology, 106*(1), 126–137.

Boniwell, I. (2012). *Positive psychology in a nutshell: The science of happiness.* Open University Press.

Breitman, B. E. (2006). Holy listening: Cultivating a hearing heart. In H. A. Addison & B. E. Breitman (Eds.), *Jewish spiritual direction: An innovative guide from traditional and contemporary sources* (pp. 73–94). Jewish Lights.

Breyer, S. G. (2020–2021). A justice and a friend. *Columbia Law Review, 121*, RBG. https://columbialawreview.org/content/a-justice-and-a-friend/

Bridges, W. (2009). *Managing transitions: Making the most of change.* DaCapo Press.

Bronfenbrenner, U. (1994). Ecological models of human development. *International Encyclopedia of Education, 3*(2), 37–43.

Brooks, A. (2022). *From strength to strength: Finding success, happiness and deep purpose in the second half of life.* Portfolio Publishing.

Brown, B. (2010). *The gifts of imperfection: Let go of who you think you're supposed to be and embrace who you are – Your guide to a wholehearted life.* Hazelden Publishing.

Brown, B. (2021). *Atlas of the heart: Mapping meaningful connection and the language of human experience.* Random House.

Brown University. (2018). *Overcome procrastination.* https://www.brown.edu/campus-life/support/counseling-and-psychological-services/index.php?q=overcoming-procrastination.

Cameron, K. (2012). *Positive leadership: Strategies for extraordinary performance.* Berrett-Koehler Publishers.

Carstensen, L. L. (2006). The influence of a sense of time on human development. *Science, 312*(5782), 1913–1915. https://www.ncbi.nlm.nih.gov/pmc/articles/PMC2790864/

Cheavens, J. S., Heiy, J. E., Feldman, D. B., Benitez, C., & Rand, K. L. (2019). Hope, goals, and pathways: Further validating the hope scale with observer ratings. *The Journal of Positive Psychology, 14*(4), 452–462.

Clear, J. (2018). *Atomic habits: An easy and proven way to build good habits and break bad ones.* Avery.

Cleveland Clinic. (2025). *Cortisol.*
https://my.clevelandclinic.org/health/articles/22187-cortisol

Cohen, R., Bavishi, C., & Rosanski, A. (2015). Purpose in life and its relationship to all-cause mortality and cardiovascular events: A meta-analysis. *Psychosomatic Medicine, 78*(2), 122–133.

Cowan, R., & Thal, L. (2015). *Wise aging: Living with joy, resilience, & spirit.* Behrman House.

Csikszentmihalyi, M. (1990). *Flow: The psychology of optimal experience.* Harper & Row.

Csikszentmihalyi, M. (1996). *Creativity: Flow and the psychology of discovery and invention.* Harper & Row.

Dalai Lama, H. H., & Cutler, H. C. (1998). *The art of happiness: A handbook for living* (10th anniversary ed.). Riverhead Books.

The Dalai Lama's 6 key tips to happiness. (2017, July 7). http://www.awaken.com/2017/07/the-dalai-lamas-6-key-tips-to-happiness/

Damon, W., Menon, J., & Bronk, K. C. (2003). The development of purpose during adolescence. *Applied Developmental Science, 7*(3), 119–128.

Dass, R., & Bush, M. (2018). *Walking each other home: Conversations on loving and dying.* Sounds True.

Diehl, M., Smyer, M. A., & Mehrotra, C. M. (2020). Optimizing aging: A call for a new narrative. *American Psychologist, 75*(4), 577–589.

Dreher, D. (2008). *Your personal renaissance: 12 steps to finding your life's true calling.* DaCapo.

Duckworth, A. (2016). *Grit: The power of passion and perseverance.* Scribner.

Duckworth, A. (2016). *Grit scale.* http://angeladuckworth.com/grit-scale/

Duckworth, A. L., Peterson, C., Matthews, M. D., & Kelly, D. R. (2007). Grit: Perseverance and passion for long-term goals. *Journal of Personality and Social Psychology, 92*(6), 1087–1101.

Duehren, A. M. (2015). To applause and admiration, Ginsburg receives Radcliffe Medal. *The Harvard Crimson.* https://www.thecrimson.com/article/2015/5/31/ ginsburg-radcliffe-medal-2015/

Dweck, C. (2006). *Mindset: The new psychology of success.* Random House.

Dweck, C. S. (2006–2010). *Mindset.* https://mindsetonline.com/changeyourmindset/firststeps/index.html

Dweck, C. (2014, December 17). *Carol Dweck: The power of believing that you can improve* [Video]. TED. https://www.ted.com/talks/carol_dweck_the_power_ of_believing_that_you_can_improve

Dweck, C. (2016). What having a "growth mindset" actually means. *Harvard Business Review.* https://hbr.org/2016/01/what-having- a-growth-mindset-actually-means

Easvaradoss, V., & Rajan, T. (2013). Positive psychology, spirituality and well-being: An overview. *Indian Journal of Positive Psychology, 4*(2), 321–325.

Egeland, B., Carlson, E., & Sroufe, L. (1993). Resilience as process. *Development and Psychopathology, 5*(4), 517–528.

Elias, M. J. (2006). The connection between academic and social-emotional learning. In M. J. Elias & H. Arnold (Eds.), *The educator's guide to emotional intelligence and academic achievement: Social-emotional learning in the classroom* (pp. 4–14). Corwin Press.

Elias, M. J., Tobias, S. E., & Friedlander, B. S. (1999). *Emotionally intelligent parenting: How to raise a self-disciplined, responsible, socially skilled child.* Harmony Books.

Ellis, A., & Harper, R. A. (1997). *A guide to rational living.* Albert Ellis Institute.

Emmons, R. A. (2007). *Thanks! How the new science of gratitude can make you happier.* Houghton Mifflin.

Emmons, R. A. (2016). *The little book of gratitude: Create a life of happiness and wellbeing by giving thanks.* Hachette Book Group.

Emmons, R. A., & McCullough, M. E. (2003). Counting blessings versus burdens: An experimental investigation of gratitude and subjective well-being in daily life. *Journal of Personality and Social Psychology, 84*(2), 377–389.

Emmons, R. A., & Mishra, A. (2012). Why gratitude enhances well-being: What we know, what we need to know. In K. Sheldon, T. Kashdan, & M. F. Steger (Eds.), *Designing the future of positive psychology: Taking stock and moving forward.* Oxford University Press.

Ericsson, K. A., Prietula, M., & Cokely, E. (2007, July). The making of an expert. *Harvard Business Review.* https://hbr.org/2007/07/the-making-of-an-expert

Erikson, E. H. (1963). *Childhood and society* (Vol. 2). Norton.

Erikson, E. H. (1968). *Identity: Youth and crisis.* W. W. Norton & Co.

Feldman, D. B., Rand, K. L., & Kahle-Wrobleski, K. (2009). Hope and goal attainment: Testing a basic premise of hope theory. *Journal of Social and Clinical Psychology, 28*(4), 479–497.

Feldman, D. B., & Dreher, D. (2011). Can hope be changed in 90 minutes? Testing the efficacy of a single-session goal-pursuit intervention for college students. *Journal of Happiness Studies, 13*, 45–59.

Flett, G. L. (2022). An introduction, review, and conceptual analysis of mattering as an essential construct and an essential way of life. *Journal of Psychoeducational Assessment, 40*(1), 3–16.

Frankl, V. (1959). *Man's search for meaning.* New York, NY: Washington Square Press.

Frankl, V. (1985). *Man's search for meaning* (Rev. & updated ed.). New York, NY: Washington Square Press.

Fredrickson, B. L. (2004). The broaden-and-build theory of positive emotions. *Philosophical Transactions of the Royal Society, 359*, 1367–1377.

Fredrickson, B. L. (2009). *Positivity: Top-notch research reveals the upward spiral that will change your life.* New York, NY: Three Rivers Press.

Fredrickson, B. L. (2013). *Love 2.0: How our supreme emotion affects everything we feel, think, do, and become.* New York, NY: Hudson Street Press.

Fredrickson, B. L. (2013). Positive emotions broaden and build. In *Advances in experimental social psychology* (Vol. 47, pp. 1–53). Academic Press.

Fredrickson, B. L. (2013). NIH Record: Fredrickson describes nourishing power of small positive moments. *LXV*(10). https://nihrecord.nih.gov/newsletters/2013/05_10_2013/story3.htm

Fredrickson, B. L. (May, 2020). *Positivity and tragedy.* Online Lunch & Learn, Marlene Meyerson JCC Manhattan & Wholebeing Institute.

Fredrickson, B. L., Tugade, M. M., Waugh, C. E., & Larkin, G. R. (2003). What good are positive emotions in crises? A prospective study of resilience and emotions following the terrorist attacks on the United States on September 11th, 2001. *Journal of Personality and Social Psychology, 84*(2), 365–376.

Friedman, H. A. Center for Aging, Washington University in St. Louis. (2021, April 22). *Realizing the potential of longer life: The new "Longevity Economy" – 2021 Friedman Lecture & Awards Summary.* https://publichealth.wustl.edu/realizing-the-potential-of-longer-life-the-new-longevity-economy/

Fulghum, R. (1986). *All I really need to know I learned in kindergarten: Uncommon thoughts on common things.* New York, NY: Villard Books.

Gendron, T. L., Welleford, E. A., Inker, J., & White, J. T. (2016). The language of ageism: Why we need to use words carefully. *The Gerontologist, 56*(6), 997–1006.

Gill, T. M., Murphy, T. E., Barry, L. C., & Allore, H. G. (2009). Risk factors for disability subtypes in older persons. *Journal of the American Geriatrics Society, 57*, 1850–1855. https://www.ncbi.nlm.nih.gov/pmc/articles/PMC2782909/pdf/nihms154895.pdf

Ginsberg, R. B. (2016, October 1). Ruth Bader Ginsburg's advice for living. *New York Times.* https://www.nytimes.com/2016/10/02/opinion/sunday/ruth-bader-ginsburgs-advice-for-living.html

Goldstein, E. (2013). Stressing out? S.T.O.P. Retrieved from https://www.mindful.org/stressing-out-stop/

Goleman, D. (1995). *Emotional intelligence: Why it can matter more than IQ.* New York, NY: Bantam Books.

Goleman, D., & Boyatzis, R. (2017). Emotional intelligence has 12 elements. Which do you need to work on? *Harvard Business Review, 84*(2), 1–5.

Goleman, D., & Davidson, R. J. (2017). *Altered traits: Science reveals how meditation changes your mind, brain, and body.* New York, NY: Avery.

Gonzales, M. (2012). *Mindful leadership: The 9 ways to self-awareness, transforming yourself, and inspiring others.* Mississauga, Ontario: Jossey-Bass.

Green, A. M. (2019). Five ways to have better conversations across difference. https://greatergood.berkeley.edu/article/item/five_ways_to_have_better_conversations_across_difference

Hays, K. (2002). *Move your body: Tone your mood.* Oakland, CA: New Harbinger.

Hays, K. (2017). The 80% edge. https://www.psychologytoday.com/us/blog/the-edge-peak-performance-psychology/201705/the-80-edge

Hays, K. (2018, July 11). Personal communication – Interview with Ilene Berns-Zare.

Hays, K. F., & Brown, C. H., Jr. (2004). *You're on! Consulting for peak performance.* Washington, DC: American Psychological Association.

Herford, R. T. (1962). *The ethics of the Talmud: Sayings of the fathers.* New York, NY: Schocken Books.

Hill, P. L., & Turiano, N. A. (2014). Purpose in life as a predictor of mortality across adulthood. *Psychological Science, 25*(7), 1482–1486. https://doi.org/10.1177/0956797614531799

Hobson, N. M., Schroeder, J., Risen, J. L., Xygalatas, D., & Inzlicht, M. (2018). The psychology of rituals: An integrative review and process-based framework. *Personality and Social Psychology Review, 22*(3), 260–284.

Jane Goodall Institute. (2025). About Jane. https://janegoodall.org/our-story/about-jane/

Johnson, A. (2021). *A model system: Resilience and performance strategies as predictors of flow state in elite three-day equestrians* (Master's thesis, Harvard University Division of Continuing Education).

Jose, P. E., Lim, B. T., & Bryant, F. B. (2012). Does savoring increase happiness? A daily diary study. *The Journal of Positive Psychology, 7*(3), 176–187.

Jung, C. G. (1971). The stages of life. In J. Campbell (Ed.), *The portable Jung* (pp. 3–22). New York, NY: Penguin Books.

Kabat-Zinn, J. (1994). *Wherever you go there you are: Mindfulness meditation in everyday life.* New York, NY: Hyperion.

Kabat-Zinn, J. (2012). *Mindfulness for beginners: Reclaiming the present moment—and your life.* Boulder, CO: Sounds True.

Kaufman, S. B. (2020). *Transcend: The new science of self-actualization.* New York, NY: TarcherPerigee.

Kellerman, G. R., & Seligman, M. (2023). *Tomorrowmind: Thriving at work with resilience, creativity, and connection—now and in an uncertain future.* New York, NY: Simon & Schuster.

Kennedy, J. J., & Gonzalez, M. (2023). How neuroplasticity affects creativity: Understanding our brain's ability to innovate. https://www.psychologytoday.com/us/blog/brain-reboot/202306/how-neuroplasticity-affects-creativity

Kessler, E. M., & Staudinger, U. M. (2007). Intergenerational potential: Effects of social interaction between older adults and adolescents. *Psychology and Aging, 22*(4), 690–704. https://doi.org/10.1037/0882-7974.22.4.690

Kouzes, J. M., & Posner, B. Z. (2011). *Credibility: How leaders gain and lose it, why people demand it.* Hoboken, NJ: John Wiley & Sons.

Krause, M. (2023). Developing mental toughness in young baseball players. https://pbsccs.org/developing-mental-toughness-in-young-baseball-players.

Langer, E. J. (2009). *Counter clockwise: Mindful health and the power of possibility.* Ballantine Books.

Layous, K., & Lyubomirsky, S. (2014). The how, why, what, when, and who of happiness: Mechanisms underlying the success of positive activity interventions. In J. Gruber & J. T. Moskowitz (Eds.), *Positive emotion: Integrating the light sides and dark sides* (pp. 473–495). Oxford University Press.

Legrand, E., Bieleke, M., Gollwitzer, P. M., & Mignon, A. (2017, April 10). *Nothing will stop me: Flexibly tenacious goal striving with implementation intentions.* https://www.researchgate.net/publication/315912581_Nothing_Will_Stop_Me_Flexibly_Tenacious_Goal_Striving_With_Implementation_Intentions

Levy, B. (2009). Stereotype embodiment: A psychosocial approach to aging. *Current Directions in Psychological Science, 18*(6), 332–336.

Levy, B. R., Slade, M. D., Kunkel, S. R., & Kasi, S. V. (2002). Longevity increased by positive self-perceptions of aging. *Journal of Personality and Social Psychology, 83*(2), 261–270.

Losada, M., & Heaphy, E. (2004). The role of positivity and connectivity in the performance of business teams: A nonlinear model. *American Behavioral Scientist, 47*(6), 740–765.

Luchetti, M., Terracciano, A., Stephan, Y., & Sutin, A. R. (2016). Personality and cognitive decline in older adults: Data from a longitudinal sample and meta-analysis. *The Journals of Gerontology: Series B, 71*(3), 591–601.

Margolius, M. (2018). Kavod: Witnessing the divine in self and other. In *Mindful Torah for our time: Meeting challenges with clarity and wisdom.* Institute for Jewish Spirituality.

Malone, J. C., Liu, S. R., Vaillant, G. E., Rentz, D. M., & Waldinger, R. J. (2016). Midlife Eriksonian psychosocial development: Setting the stage for late-life cognitive and emotional health. *Developmental Psychology, 52*(3), 496–505.

Martela, F., Laitinen, E., & Hakulinen, C. (2024). Which predicts longevity better: Satisfaction with life or purpose in life? *Psychology and Aging, 29*(6).

Maslow, A. H. (1943). A theory of human motivation. *Psychological Review, 50*(4), 370–396.

Maslow, A. H. (1987). *Motivation and personality* (3rd ed.). Harper & Row.

Mather, M., & Carstensen, L. L. (2005). Aging and motivated cognition: The positivity effect in attention and memory. *Trends in Cognitive Sciences, 9*(10), 496–502.

Matta, C., & Jacobsen, J. (2025, July 7). *Resilience: Mindfulness and Flow.* Retrieved from https://www.mentalhealth.com/library/resilience-mindfulness-and-flow.

McKnight, P. E., & Kashdan, T. B. (2009). Purpose in life as a system that creates and sustains health and well-being: An integrative, testable theory. *Review of General Psychology, 13*(3), 242–251.

Miskovic, V., & Lynn, S. J. (2025). *Dreaming reality: How neuroscience and mysticism can unlock the secrets of consciousness.* The Belknap Press of Harvard University Press.

Moore, M., Jackson, E., & Tschannen-Moran, B. (2016). *Coaching psychology manual* (2nd ed.). Wolters Kluwer.

Naor, L. (2016). Peak experience: When flow gains meaning. *Positive Living Newsletter.* http://www.drpaulwong.com/peak-experience/

Neff, K. (2011). *Self-compassion: The proven power of being kind to yourself.* William Morrow.

Neff, K., & Germer, C. (2018). *The mindful self-compassion workbook: A proven way to accept yourself, build inner strength, and thrive.* Guilford Press.

Neff, K., & Germer, C. (2019). The transformative effects of mindful self-compassion. https://www.mindful.org/the-transformative-effects-of-mindful-self-compassion/

Newberry, L. (2023). What we're missing out on when we don't have intergenerational relationships, personally and professionally. *Los Angeles Times.* https://www.latimes.com/california/newsletter/ 2023-04-11/what-were-missing-out-on-when-we- dont-have-intergenerational-relationships-personally -and-collectively-group-therapy

Niemiec, R. M. (2014). *Mindfulness & character strengths: A practical guide to flourishing.* Hogrefe Publishing.

Niemiec, R. M. (2018). *Character strengths interventions: A field guide for practitioners.* Hogrefe.

Norton, M. (2024). *The ritual effect: From habit to ritual, harness the surprising power of everyday actions.* Scribner.

Oettingen, G. (2014). *Rethinking positive thinking: Inside the new science of motivation.* Current Publishing.

Oettingen, G. (2024). WOOP. https://woopmylife.org/en/practice

Oettingen, G., & Gollwitzer, P. M. (2010). Strategies of setting and implementing goals: Mental contrasting and implementation intention. In J. E. Maddux & J. P. Tangney (Eds.), *Social psychological foundations of clinical psychology* (pp. 114–136). Guilford Press.

Oliver, M. (2017). *Devotions: The selected poems of Mary Oliver.* Penguin Books.

Palmer, P. (2024). *A hidden wholeness: The journey toward an undivided life – Welcoming the soul and weaving community in a wounded world.* John Wiley & Sons.

Pagnini, F., Cavalera, C., Volpato, E., Comazzi, B., Vailate Riboni, F., Valota, C., Bercovitz, K., Molinari, E., Banfi, P., Phillips, D., & Langer, E. (2019). Aging as a mindset: A study protocol to rejuvenate older adults with a counterclockwise psychological intervention. *BMJ Open, 9*(7).

Pennebaker, J. W., & Smyth, J. M. (2016). *Opening up by writing it down: How expressive writing improves health and eases emotional pain.* The Guilford Press.

Peterson, C. (2006). *A primer in positive psychology.* Oxford University Press.

Peterson, C. (2008). What is positive psychology, and what is it not? Positive psychology studies what makes life most worth living. https://www.psychologytoday.com/us/blog/the-good-life/200805/what-is-positive-psychology-and-what-is-it-not

Peterson, C., & Seligman, M. E. P. (2004). *Character strengths and virtues: A handbook and classification.* American Psychological Association.

Ponte, D. V., & Schäfer, L. (2013). Carl Gustav Jung, quantum physics and the spiritual mind: A mystical vision of the twenty-first century. *Behavioral Sciences, 3*(4), 601–618. https://doi.org/10.3390/bs3040601

Posluns, K., & Gall, T. L. (2020). Dear mental health practitioners, take care of yourselves: A literature review on self-care. *International Journal for the Advancement of Counselling, 42*(1), 1–20.

Prochaska, J. O., Norcross, J. C., & DiClemente, C. O. (1994). *Changing for good: A revolutionary six-stage program for overcoming bad habits and moving your life positively forward.* HarperCollins.

Pychyl, T. A. (2010). *Solving the procrastination puzzle: A concise guide to strategies for change.* Penguin Group.

Ramachandran, V. S. (2011). *The tell-tale brain: A neuroscientist's quest for what makes us human*. W. W. Norton & Co.

Rand, K. L., & Cheavens, J. S. (2009). *Hope theory*. In S. J. Lopez & C. R. Snyder (Eds.), *The Oxford handbook of positive psychology* (pp. 323–333). Oxford University Press.

Richards, R. (n.d.). Everyday creativity: Process and way of life – Four key issues (pp. 189–215). https://doi.org/10.1017/CBO9780511763205.013

Richards, R. (2007). Everyday creativity: Our hidden potential. In R. Richards (Ed.), *Everyday creativity and new views of human nature: Psychological, social, and spiritual perspectives* (pp. 25–53). American Psychological Association.

Rizzolatti, G., Fabbri-Destro, M., & Cattaneo, L. (2009). Mirror neurons and their clinical relevance. *Nature clinical practice neurology, 5*(1), 24-34.

Rogers, C. R. (1961). *On becoming a person*. Houghton Mifflin.

Rogers, C. R. (1995). *On becoming a person: A therapist's view of psychotherapy*. Houghton Mifflin Harcourt.

Roth, L. H. O., & Laireiter, A. R. (2021). Factor structure of the "Top Ten" positive emotions of Barbara Fredrickson. *Frontiers in Psychology, 12*, 641804. https://doi.org/10.3389/fpsyg.2021.641804

Rumi, J. A. D., & Barks, C. (1995). *The essential Rumi*. HarperCollins.

Rutter, M. (1993). Resilience: Some conceptual considerations. *Journal of Adolescent Health, 14*, 626–631.

Salzberg, S. (2014). *Real happiness at work: Meditations for accomplishment, achievement, and peace*. Workman Publishing.

Schechter-Shalomi, Z., & Miller, R. (1995). *From age-ing to sage-ing: A revolutionary approach to growing older.* Grand Central Publishing.

Scherer, K. R., Schorr, A., & Johnstone, T. (Eds.). (2001). *Appraisal processes in emotion: Theory, methods, research.* Oxford University Press.

Seligman, M. E. P. (2002). *Authentic happiness: Using the new positive psychology to realize your potential for lasting fulfillment.* Atria Paperbacks.

Seligman, M. E. P. (2011). *Flourish: A visionary new understanding of happiness and well-being.* Atria Paperback.

Seligman, M. E. P., & Csikszentmihalyi, M. (2000). Positive psychology: An introduction. *American Psychologist, 55*(1), 5–14.

Seligman, M. E. P., Steen, T. A., Park, N., & Peterson, C. (2005). Positive psychology progress: Empirical validation of interventions. *American Psychologist, 60*(5), 410–421. https://doi.org/10.1037/0003-066X.60.5.410

Shapiro, S. L., Brown, K. W., & Biegel, G. M. (2007). Teaching self-care to caregivers: Effects of mindfulness-based stress reduction on the mental health of therapists in training. *Training and Education in Professional Psychology, 1*(2), 105–115. https://doi.org/10.1037/1931-3918.1.2.105

Sheldon, K. (2004). *Optimal human being: An integrated multi-level perspective.* Lawrence Erlbaum Associates.

Shonin, E., Van Gordon, W., & Griffiths, M. D. (2015). Does mindfulness work? *BMJ, 351.* https://doi.org/10.1136/bmj.h6919

Siegel, D. (2011). *Mindsight: The new science of personal transformation.* Bantam Books.

Siegel, D. (2012). *Pocket guide to interpersonal neurobiology: An integrative handbook of the mind.* W. W. Norton & Co.

Simonton, D. K. (2001). Creativity. In C. R. Snyder & S. J. Lopez (Eds.), Handbook of positive psychology (pp. 189-201). Oxford University Press.

Sinek, S. (2009). *Start with why: How great leaders inspire everyone to take action*. Penguin Group.

Smith, C. A., & Lazarus, R. S. (1991). Emotion and adaptation. In L. A. Pervin (Ed.), *Handbook of personality: Theory and research* (pp. 609–637). Guilford Press.

Smith, J. L., & Hollinger-Smith, L. (2015). Savoring, resilience, and psychological well-being in older adults. *Aging & Mental Health, 19*(3), 192–200. https://doi.org/10.1080/13607863.2014.986647

Smith, A. C., & Stewart, B. (2011). Organizational rituals: Features, functions and mechanisms. *International Journal of Management Reviews, 13*(2), 113–133. https://doi.org/10.1111/j.1468-2370.2010.00288.x

Snyder, C. R. (1994). *The psychology of hope*. Free Press.

Snyder, C. R. (Ed.). (2000). *Handbook of hope: Theory, measures, and applications*. Academic Press.

Snyder, C. R., Rand, K. L., & Sigmon, D. R. (2002). Hope theory: A member of the positive psychology family. In C. R. Snyder & S. J. Lopez (Eds.), *The handbook of positive psychology* (pp. 257–275). Oxford University Press.

Stanford Center on Longevity. (2016). *Hidden in plain sight: How intergenerational relationships can transform our future.* https://longevity.stanford.edu/wp-content/uploads/2017/04/Monograph_web_07_11_2016.pdf

Stanford University Center for Teaching and Learning. (2025). *Top 10 learning strategies.* https://studentlearning.stanford.edu/top-10-learning-strategies

Staudinger, U. M. (2001). Life reflection: A social-cognitive analysis of life review. *Review of General Psychology, 5*(2), 148–160.

Staudinger, U. M. (2020). The positive plasticity of adult development: Potential for the 21st century. *American Psychologist, 75*(4), 540–553.

Sternberg, E. M. (2001). *The balance within: The science connecting health and emotions.* W. H. Freeman.

Stewart, A. J., & Vandewater, E. A. (1999). "If I had it to do over again …": Midlife review, midcourse corrections, and women's well-being in midlife. *Journal of Personality and Social Psychology, 76*(2), 270–283.

Stone, B. M., & Parks, A. C. (2018). Cultivating subjective well-being through positive psychological interventions. In E. Diener, S. Oishi, & L. Tay (Eds.), *Handbook of well-being.* DEF Publishers.

Swimme, B., & Berry, T. (1992). *The universe story: From the primordial flaring forth to the ecozoic era – A celebration of the unfolding of the cosmos.* HarperCollins Publishers.

Ter Kuile, C. (2020). *The power of ritual: Turning everyday activities into soulful practices.* Harper One.

Thakar, V. (1984). *Spirituality and social action: A holistic approach.* Vimala Programs.

Tucker-Drob, E. M., & Briley, D. A. (2014). Continuity of genetic and environmental influences on cognition across the life span: A meta-analysis of longitudinal twin and adoption studies. *Psychological Bulletin, 140*(4), 949–979. https://doi.org/10.1037/a0035893

Tyler, A. L. (2020–2021). Lessons learned from Justice Ruth Bader Ginsburg. *Columbia Law Review, 121*(RBG). https://columbialawreview.org/content/lessons-learned-from-justice-ruth-bader-ginsburg/

U.S. Census Bureau. (n.d.). *Population projections.* Retrieved October 25, 2019, from
https://www.census.gov/programs-surveys/popproj.html

University of Washington School of Medicine, Institute for Health Metrics and Evaluation. (2024, March 11). *COVID-19 had greater impact on life expectancy than previously known, but child mortality rates continued to decline during the pandemic.*
https://www.healthdata.org/news-events/newsroom/news-releases/covid-19-had-greater-impact-life-expectancy-previously-known

Vaillant, G. E. (2003). *Aging well: Surprising guideposts to a happier life from the landmark Harvard study of adult development.* Little, Brown & Company.

VIA Institute on Character. (n.d.). *The VIA classification of character strengths and virtues.*
https://www.viacharacter.org/www/Character-Strengths/VIA-Classification

Waldinger, R. J. (2004). *The Harvard Study on Adult Development.*
http://hr1973.org/docs/Harvard35thReunion_Waldinger.pdf

Waldinger, R. J. (2015, November). *What makes a good life: Lessons from the longest study on happiness* [TED Talk]. https://www.ted.com/talks/robert_waldinger_what_makes_a_good_life_lessons_from_the_longest_study_on_happiness

Waldinger, R. (2022). *TED – 7 years later: Harvard Study of Adult Development.* https://www.adultdevelopmentstudy.org/

Warren, R., Smeets, E., & Neff, K. (2016). Risk and resilience: Being compassionate to oneself is associated with emotional resilience and psychological well-being. *Current Psychiatry, 15*(2), 19–33.

Waters, L. (2017). *The strengths switch: How the science of strength-based parenting can help your child and your teen to flourish.* Penguin Random House.

Welcome to the Harvard Study of Adult Development. (2015). https://www.adultdevelopmentstudy.org/

Werner, E. (1994). Overcoming the odds. *Developmental and Behavioral Pediatrics, 15*(2), 131–136.

Willard, C. (2016). *Growing up mindful: Essential practices to help children, teens, and families find balance, calm, and resilience.* Sounds True.

Williams, M., & Penman, D. (2011). *Mindfulness: An eight-week plan for finding peace in a frantic world.* Rodale Press.

Wilson, C. A., & Saklofske, D. H. (2018). The relationship between trait emotional intelligence, resiliency, and mental health in older adults: The mediating role of savoring. *Aging & Mental Health*, 22(5), 646–654.

Wong, P. T. (2016). Meaning-seeking, self-transcendence, and well-being. In A. Batthyany (Ed.), *Logotherapy and existential analysis: Proceedings of the Viktor Frankl Institute* (Vol. 1, pp. 311–322). Springer International Publishing.

Zagano, P., & Gillespie, C. K. (2006). Ignatian spirituality and positive psychology. *The Way, 45*(4), 41–58.

Zimmerman, G. L., Olsen, C. G., & Bosworth, M. F. (2000). A "states of change" approach to helping patients change behavior. *American Family Physician, 61*(5), 1409–1414.

www.ingramcontent.com/pod-product-compliance
Lightning Source LLC
Chambersburg PA
CBHW062211270326
41930CB00009B/1707